Disciplining Birth

DISCIPLINING BIRTH
Power, Knowledge and Childbirth
Practices in Bangladesh

Kaosar Afsana

The University Press Limited

The University Press Limited
Red Crescent House
61 Motijheel C/A
P. O. Box 2611
Dhaka 1000
Bangladesh
Fax : (88 02) 9565443
E-mail: upl@bangla.net
Website: www.uplbooks.com

First published 2005

Copyright © The University Press Limited

All rights are reserved. No part of this publication may be reproduced or transmitted in any form or by any means without prior permission in writing from the publisher. Any person who does any unauthorised act in relation to this publication may be liable to criminal prosecution and civil claims for damages.

Cover design by Ashraful Hassan Arif

ISBN 984 05 1741 4

Published by Mohiuddin Ahmed, The University Press Limited, Dhaka. Computer design by Ashim K. Biswas and produce by Abortan, 99 Malibagh, Dhaka. Printed at Akata Offset Press, 119 Fakirapool, Dhaka, Bangladesh.

To
mothers, sisters and daughters

Contents

List of Photographs ix
Acronyms xi
Acknowledgements xiii
Preface xv

Chapter 1
Situating Childbirth 1
    1.1 Birth: Evolution of the Problem 2
    1.2 Research Methods and Concerns 8
    1.3 Organisation of Birth Experiences in Bangladesh 11

Chapter 2
The Research Scene 15
    2.1 The Village of *Apurbabari* 15
    2.2 The Thana Health Complex 20
    2.3 The Medical College Hospital 24
    2.4 Summary and Conclusion 29

Chapter 3
Two Contemporary Birth Practices:
Observational Experiences 31
    3.1 Indigenous Birthing Care 32
    3.2 Arrival of Cosmopolitan Obstetrics 45
    3.3 Summary and Conclusion 58

Chapter 4
Indigenous Birth Practices: Construction of Birth in *Apurbabari* 63
    4.1 Women in Birthing 63
    4.2 Indigenous Knowledge: The Role of *Dainis* 86

	4.3	Where are Men ?	99
	4.4	Local Healers and Health Practitioners	101
	4.5	Summary and Conclusion	107

Chapter 5
Cosmopolitan Obstetrics: Construction of Birth in Hospitals — 111

	5.1	Embodied Feeling of being a Doctor	112
	5.2	Meeting Doctors in the Hospital	112
	5.3	My Immediate Experiences in the Hospital	113
	5.4	Experiencing Hospital: Women and their Families	115
	5.5	Doctors in Cosmopolitan Obstetrics	141
	5.6	Nurses Attending Wards	149
	5.7	Special *Ayah's* Experiences: Silent Sufferings	153
	5.8	Cosmopolitan Obstetrics in Village Landscape	155
	5.9	Summary and Conclusion	157

Chapter 6
Anatomies of Birth — 161

	6.1	Construction of Birth: Limits of Plurality	162
	6.2	Embodied Knowledge and Engagement in Birth	165
	6.3	Women's Silence: Home and the World	169
	6.4	Indigenous Knowledge of Birth: The Role of *Dainis*	172
	6.5	Marginalisation of Indigenous Knowledge	178
	6.6	Hospital: Power of Design and Space	181
	6.7	Authoritative Knowledge of Biomedical Professionals	183
	6.8	The Triad: Doctor, Nurse and Patient	187
	6.9	Fiscal Violence	191
	6.10	Women, State and Obstetric Care	195
	6.11	Summary and Conclusion	200

Chapter 7
Epilogue and the Future — 203

	7.1	This Research and the Signification	205
	7.2	Future Research Sketch	207
	7.3	What Changes can be Made in Future Birth	209

References — 219

Index — 235

List of Photographs

Photo 1	: A village hut	36
Photo 2	: Raheemon sat in the courtyard in front of Taljan's hut	36
Photo 3	: In THC labour room, a birthing woman was surrounded by relatives	49
Photo 4	: The THC labour room	49
Photo 5	: In the THC, a husband stood beside his wife's bed	50
Photo 6	: Patients' attendants were waiting in hospital corridor	56
Photo 7	: A doctor was examining a patient in a postnatal ward	57
Photo 8	: Hashima was grinding spices the day before her labour pain	67
Photo 9	: Ambika was giving bath to Raheemon's newborn baby, and Taljan, the *daini* was watching the event along with the neighbours	67
Photo 10	: A mother-in-law was helping the first-time mother breastfeed the baby. A *daini* sat beside them	77
Photo 11	: Hashima was massaging the newborn baby with oil in *chodighar*	78
Photo 12	: A baby was seen to be protected from evil spirits and evil winds by placing a broom, a leather sandal and a sickle	79
Photo 13	: A barber was shaving a newborn baby's hair on the seventh day to remove pollution	80
Photo 14	: The Medical College Hospital obstetric ward	128
Photo 15	: The Medical College Hospital labour room	129

Acronyms

AHI	Assistant Health Inspector
ANC	Antenatal Care
BIRPERHT	Bangladesh Institute of Research for Promotion of Essential & Reproductive Health and Technologies
BRAC	Bangladesh Rural Advancement Committee
BHC	BRAC Health Centre
CHW	Community Health Worker
DGFP	Directorate General of Family Planning
DGHS	Directorate General of Health Services
DNS	Directorate of Nursing Services
EOC	Emergency Obstetric Care
EPI	Expanded Program on Immunization
EsOC	Essential Obstetric Care
FWA	Family Welfare Assistant
FWV	Family Welfare Visitor
HA	Health Assistant
HPSP	Health and Population Sector Program
ICDDR,B	International Centre for Diarrhoeal Disease Research, Bangladesh.
MOHFW	Ministry of Health and Family Welfare
MO-MCH	Medical Officer-Maternal and Child Health
NIPORT	National Institute for Population Research and Training
RMO	Residential Medical Officer
RMP	Rural Medical Practitioners
SMIs	Safe Motherhood Initiatives
TBA	Traditional Birth Attendant

TFPO	Thana Family Planning Officer
THA	Thana Health Administrator
THC	Thana Health Complex
WHO	World Health Organisation
UHFWC	Union Health and Family Welfare Centre

Acknowledgements

In the last three years many people assisted me in various ways and have contributed to the development of this dissertation. First I would like to express my gratitude to the members of my supervisory team, Dr. Lynne Hunt and Dr. Nancy Hudson-Rodd, Edith Cowan University. Special thanks are due to Lynne for her insightful advice, and continual encouragement and support. I am grateful to Nancy for her advice and guidance in further organising the thesis. I am also appreciative of their warmth and hospitality during my stay at Perth.

I would like to extend my thanks to those who participated in my research. The arguments in the dissertation were made possible due to their openness, trust and hospitality.

BRAC's assistance during my fieldwork proved invaluable. I would like to acknowledge encouragement and support of Mr. Fazle Hasan Abed and Dr. AMR Chowdhury, BRAC. Special thanks are due to Ms. Sharmin Rahman Nipu for her assistance in my fieldwork. I am also appreciative of Mr. Mizanur Rahman's assistance in this regard. BRAC's program staff's hospitality is also acknowledged.

I take this opportunity to thank the International Postgraduate Research Fellowship and Edith Cowan University for providing my scholarship, without which it would have been difficult for me to pursue my studies in Australia. I also appreciate the support of Professor Linda Kristjanson, Research and Higher Degrees, Edith Cowan University. I am grateful to all the staff of Edith Cowan University who assisted me at various points.

Above all, I wish to acknowledge love and generous support of my family, especially my mother, Ms. Amina Begum and two brothers, Mr. Asaduzzaman Noor and Prof. Ahaduzamman Md. Ali. A million kisses to my beloved son, Shakil Ahmed for his love and patience and technical support in organising the pictures in the text. Finally, I would like to thank a very special person in my life – my husband, Prof. Imtiaz Ahmed for his love, encouragement and advice throughout the period.

Preface

My philosophical engagement with three women – Majeda, Kamla and Brigette encourages me to explore the world of birth. And then, many more women teach me to understand and feel this world through and inside women's voice and silence. More I try to understand, more I discover how women are caught in the politics of birth and the politics of development.

This book is about birth practices and about power and knowledge. When I recall my days in *Apurbabari* village and the adjacent Thana Health Complex and the Medical College Hospital, I envisage the events like snapshots one after another, and listen to multiple voices, but, most of all, those of the women. My experiential knowledge and analyses of the two contemporary birthing systems uncover why and in what ways rural, poor women in Bangladesh adhere to indigenous birth practices and concurrently, resist cosmopolitan obstetrics.

I have argued that understanding of birth, silence in birth, mind/body unification and embodied knowledge produced in discursive practices persuade women to adhere to indigenous birth practices. Yet, the unfixity of birth meaning makes women undecided about seeking medical care even in their birth crisis. At times, this leads to fatal consequences. This situation is worsened by women's silence causing more suffering in birth experience. On the other hand, uncertain consequences of birth lead women to search for different options of care.

Indigenous knowledge of birth is a communal knowledge, in which each woman participates and mutually exchanges knowledge. Although, birthing women actively engage themselves in birth events, *dainis* (village birth attendants) with indigenous skills provide them with physical, emotional and psychological supports. This supportive relationship between women and *dainis* is based neither on a hierarchy of knowledge nor on materialistic gain. In contrast, the interpersonal relationship among women, doctors and nurses is predicated on monopolistic, medical knowledge and professional hierarchies exacerbated by materialistic values. Despite the supportive relationship existing between *dainis* and women, indigenous knowledge of birth is challenged by cosmopolitan obstetric practices supported by the modern State. Not only is the knowledge of *dainis* marginalised, but they themselves also become apprehensive of their role in birthing care and suffer from an identity crisis on the brink of modernity.

Authoritative, biomedical knowledge is monopolistic. It situates itself at the zenith of modernity with medical dominance and denies space for the existence of other forms of knowledge. Women's embodied knowledge of birth is precluded by the dominant, authoritative knowledge of modern obstetrics. In facing modern, birthing care, they become inactive accomplices in their own birth experiences and remain silent with further physical and psychological sufferings.

Colossal hospital architecture and urban proclivity harmonize with the flourishing of biomedical professions. The grandness of hospitals does not mean that the quality of services is good. Maldistribution of resources and corrupt practices give rise to poor quality services in Bangladeshi hospitals. As a result, poor women, already incapacitated by poverty, are trapped in further poverty caused by fiscal violence incurred in hospital obstetric treatment.

The State is modern. It patronizes medical professions because its philosophy coincides with that of modern biomedicine, which is based on scientific rationalism, technology, capitalism and patriarchy. Despite the roots of maternal mortality and morbidity being embedded in socio-economic causes, the health policy and planning geared to a medical model of health care facilitates medical professions and hence, medicalisation of childbirth.

It is not my contention to compare and contrast these two polarised birthing systems. I present experiences from two systems in order to highlight the strengths and limitations of each. My research demonstrates that rural, poor women do adhere to indigenous birth practices and, they do resist cosmopolitan obstetrics. I have argued that that nurtured in indigenous ways of living, rural women seek assistance from indigenous birthing care because their visions and versions are similar. These women are distant from cosmopolitan obstetrics because the latter is tied up with diametrically opposed, knowledge of birth, elitism and monetary values. Although, modern biomedicine saves some lives, rural, poor women become the victim of physical, psychological, fiscal and political violence in seeking cosmopolitan obstetric care. A Foucauldian perspective has revealed the layered structures of power enforcing poor women's silence and working in consent to maintain a hierarchical, modern, medical system to the detriment of individual woman's lives and to the loss of diversity of health knowledge. These stories are told and retold, and analysed and debated, in order to ensure good health and health care for rural, poor women in Bangladesh during their birth events.

Dated: Dhaka Kaosar Afsana
August 2005

Map of Bangladesh

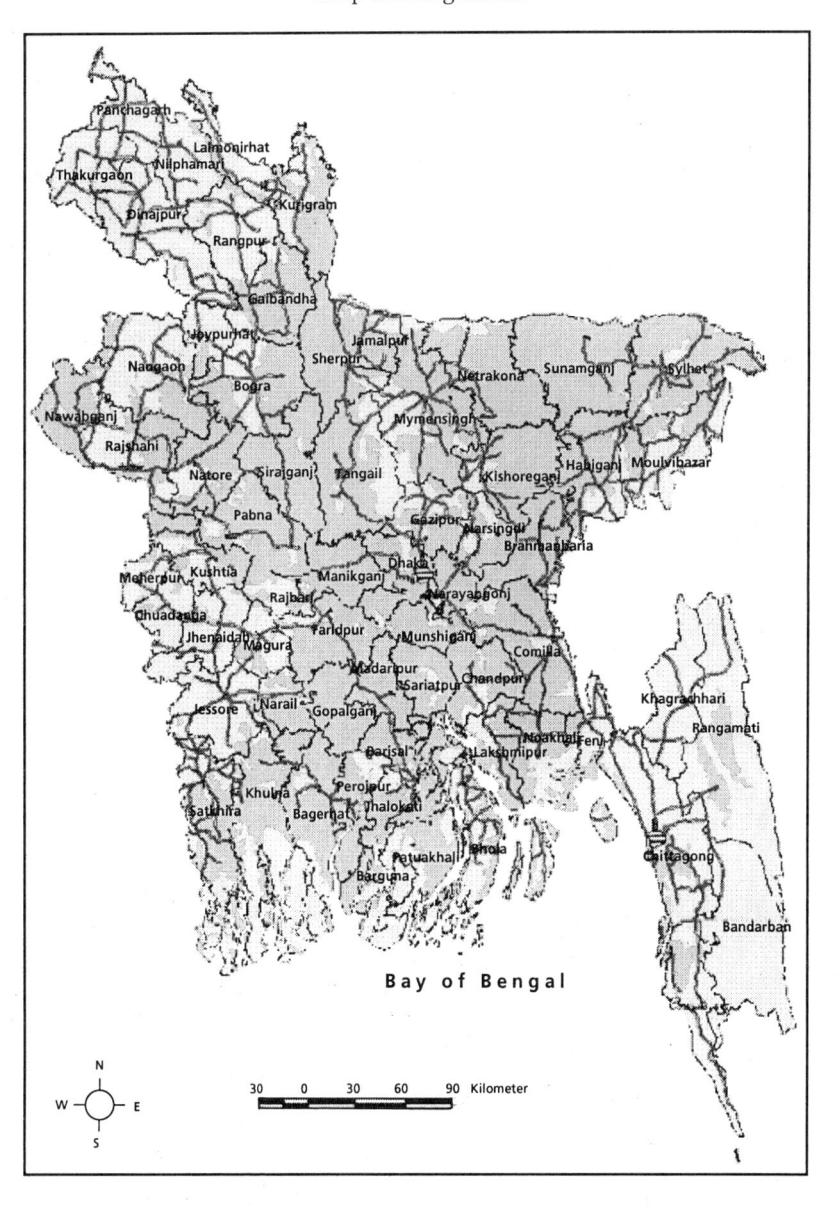

Chapter 1

Situating Childbirth

> To understand the meaning of birth
> and death we must look for
> dynamic interactions
> between physiology, society and culture.
> – Sheila Kitzinger, 1982, p. 200.

Childbirth is not only a physiological phenomenon. It is a domain where the physiology of birth is shaped and patterned by social and cultural values, not to mention the politics of birth (Davis-Floyd, 1992, 1994; Jordan, 1983, 1989; Kay, 1982; Kitzinger, 1982; MacCormack, 1982; O'Neil & Kaufert, 1990; Rothman, 1982; Sargent, 1990). While situating birth in social milieux, it is seen to be embraced by what Foucault (1978) terms "power relations" (p. 94) where interplay among different individuals, groups and social apparatus influences the construction of birth and, hence, the women's use of birthing care. In the light of this background theory and research, this study will explore birth practices among rural, poor women in Bangladesh.

To improve maternal health in Bangladesh, the government and non-governmental organisations (NGOs) with the support of international organisations offer maternity care separately and jointly as well. Nevertheless, service utilisation as yet is very poor (Bangladesh Fourth Population and Health Project, 1999; Ministry of Health and Family Welfare, 1998a; Quaiyum, Ahmed, Islam, & Khanum, 1999). Despite a number of studies exploring the complex issues of birth practices (Afsana & Rashid, 2000; Blanchet, 1984; Leppard, 2000; Rozario, 1998), there remains a paucity of information about the wide use of indigenous birthing care. Further, little is understood about rural women's reluctance to use cosmopolitan obstetric or modern obstetric care. Even so, simple quantitative or even ethnographic data cannot respond to this complex issue. To develop a wider understanding, a broad framework is required where the birthing world is analysed in its social, cultural, economic, historical and political contexts. It is this approach I have used to analyse birth practices in Bangladesh. This study has both theoretical and practical significance because information will be shared with health planners and policy-makers, health care practitioners, women, feminists, academics and the wider community to improve birthing care for rural, poor women.

1.1 BIRTH: EVOLUTION OF THE PROBLEM

My memories take me back to my childhood. It was very early in the morning when I heard some whispering voices. My mother was not in bed. She came back after a while and told my father that Majeda[1] had started her labour pains. I became very excited and wanted to see the baby right away. When daylight showed off, I ran with my little cousin to their house. I was surprised to see Majeda standing outside her thatched hut in front of the door as if waiting to greet us. I asked, "Didn't you give birth to a baby?" "Yes, I did." "Then, what are you doing here?" I asked, even more astonished. She said, "I just finished cleaning myself. I had to smear the floor with clay where the baby was born. Please go inside the room and see the baby." I entered the room and saw the baby lying on a floor-bed. Being a young girl of ten years, many questions were raised in my mind as to why she was not taking rest; why she had to clean everything; why the baby was lying on the floor; and where the other people had gone. I was interested to know more about her, but a ten-year *Bangalee* (Bengali) girl was not expected to ask questions about a birth event. I kept quiet. Much later, I came to know from Majeda that her mother-in-law and sister-in-law assisted in her birth event. They all went to work after removing the birth substances and left the other tasks for Majeda to do.

I still cannot forget the deaths of pregnant women in maternity wards during my internship in the Medical College Hospital. I still cannot forget the cry of Kamla, who begged doctors to see her. It happened in 1983 during my internship in a teaching hospital of Bangladesh. It was a very busy admission night in the Obstetric and Gynaecology unit. Two intern doctors attended pregnant women in the labour wards. The antenatal examination room was full of 10 to 12 labouring women. The clinical assistant to the unit left the ward after examining a few patients. New intern doctors became exhausted working long hours. Deliveries took place incessantly, one after the other, throughout the early morning. Kamla, a young primigravida woman, was also admitted. On examination, the doctors found that the foetal head was not engaged and Kamla's cervix was partially dilated, but she had severe abdominal pain. They advised her to be patient and went back to other patients. Kamla requested them every now and then, "*Apa* (sister), please come to me. I cannot bear my pain anymore." The intern doctors measured her blood pressure, but did not touch her abdomen, and consoled her again. Late in the morning just before the visiting of senior doctors, they prepared history and treatment sheets for each patient. Kamla seemed asleep. The clinical assistant congratulated the intern doctors for their tremendous work in managing patients successfully. When the senior doctor came to attend the patients, Kamla was found dead. The doctor said, "It's a case of ruptured uterus. She had obstructed labour." Everyone just kept quiet and then, moved to see other patients. I was extremely shocked of her death. This young lady came to the hospital for better care, but died unnoticed and undiagnosed.

I never stop thinking about Majeda's birth experience at home and Kamla's death in the hospital in giving birth to their first child. These images of Majeda and Kamla persuaded me to think and reflect on childbirth practices. The more I question myself, the more I feel that there is a need to explore childbirth practices for poor, rural women. The more I become acquainted with childbirth writings and empirical knowledge, the more I am triggered by their experiences. Who was Majeda standing so bravely just after her first birthing experience? Where did she get so much courage and strength? Was she applauded for her bravery like Ju/'huan women in Africa? Who assisted in her birth? Was her embodied knowledge of childbirth valued? Or was she a woman bequeathed with birth pollution? Concurrently, the entire incidence of Kamla's death also leaves many unresolved questions in my mind. Why did she develop obstructed labour? Was it due to her poor socio-economic status? Did she ever have antenatal care? How did she come to the hospital? Did she die due to the negligence of doctors or the overburdening of junior doctors? Why were junior doctors given so much responsibility? Was she neglected because of her poor socio-economic condition? Why did doctors remain silent about her death?

The book that deeply engages me in reflecting on indigenous childbirth practices and cosmopolitan obstetrics is Brigitte Jordan's

Birth in Four Cultures (1983). I situate Majeda and Kamla's experiences in the diverse experiences of childbirth in the four cultures. Like other scholars, Jordan recognises how the cultural specificity of social environment shapes the universality of human biology embedded in childbirth experiences. By comparing Mayan indigenous birth practices in Mexico with the cosmopolitan obstetrical practices in the United States, Holland and Sweden, Jordan feels the need to integrate indigenous and cosmopolitan birthing systems in order to improve maternal and child health in developing countries. The process of my thinking is triggered by her understandings of birth, sensitivity to indigenous knowledge, and more importantly, concept of integration about mutual exchange of knowledge between two birthing systems. The more I ponder Jordan's (1983) biosocial framework, the more I feel that the biological function of childbirth is shaped not only by socio-cultural influences but also by the political matrices of a society. Further research of Jordan (1989) looks into the cosmopolitical authority of cosmopolitan obstetrics that marginalises the indigenous knowledge of traditional midwives. The work of Chawla (2002), Davis-Floyd (1992), Kaufert (1990), Kitzinger (1982), Martin (1989), O'Neil (1990), Oakley (1984), Ram (2001), Rothman (1982), Sargent (1989), Tew (1990) and others motivates me to look into deeper issues of birth. My inspiration to do this research is instigated by the lived experiences of Majeda and Kamla, and the empirical experiences of Brigitte Jordan and many other scholars.

Majeda and Kamla were born in a country where the state of maternal health is extremely poor. The maternal mortality ratio of 600 per 100,000 live births found in community studies of Bangladesh in the early eighties (Alauddin, 1986; Khan, Jahan & Begum, 1986) declined to 320 per 100,000 live births at the beginning of the twenty-first century (National Institute for Population Research and Training, 2002). Maternal morbidity is also very high, as many as 67 episodes occur for every maternal death (Koblinsky, Campbell, & Harlow, 1993). Each year approximately four million women become pregnant and an estimated 600,000 develop complications (Ministry of Health and Family Welfare, 1998b). It is estimated that 15 percent of pregnant women require life-saving obstetric services, known as Essential Obstetric Care (EsOC). About eight percent of total births take place in different medical institutions and 2.23 percent undergo caesarean sections (Khan, Kanam, Nahar, Nasrin, & Rahman, 2000). The high infant and child mortality causes short birth intervals, which are likely to enhance women's chances of facing high maternal mortality and morbidity (Mitra, Ali, Islam, Cross & Saha, 1994). This is the scenario of maternal health in Bangladesh, a country once known as *'sonar Bangla'* – golden Bengal.

Bangladesh is situated in Southern Asia with a population of more than 128 million living in 144,000 square kilometres (Bangladesh Bureau of Statistics, 2000). It is primarily an agrarian society with a per capita income of US$ 370 per annum and a very slow economic growth of over five percent (Bangladesh Bureau of Statistics, 2000; World Bank Report, 2003). At least 70 million people live in absolute poverty, of whom women are the most disadvantaged. Anaemia, a good marker of socio-economic status and malnourishment, is prevalent among 85 percent of women and 71 percent of men at national level (Jahan & Hossain, 1998). The literacy rate for women is around 25 percent, half of male literacy rates, with an unequal distribution between urban and rural areas (Bangladesh Bureau of Statistics, 2000). The resources allocated for public health sectors are not more than five percent of the total budget (Ministry of Finance, 2002). The government expenditure for health is about US$3 per person per year, while it is estimated that US$12 is required to provide minimum level of health care to each person (Ministry of Health and Family Welfare, 1998c). Poor economic conditions, education and health care contribute to the persistently poor maternal health status.

In this pluralistic society, rural, poor women essentially access indigenous birthing care, but also seek cosmopolitan obstetric care. In indigenous practices, birth is mostly assisted by Traditional Birth Attendants (TBAs) and female relatives, and occasionally self-assisted (Afsana & Mahmud, 1998; Bangladesh Bureau of Statistics, 1999). Facilities for comprehensive obstetric services are not evenly distributed or easily accessible in rural areas. The government health facilities are hierarchically distributed in various administrative units throughout the country under the auspices of their own administration and management. They include Union Health and Family Welfare Centre (UHFWC), Thana Health Complex (THC), District Hospital (DH) and Medical College Hospital (MCH). Maternal and Child Welfare Centres (MCWCs) are sparsely located in some administrative units providing only maternity care. The activities of the government are supplemented and complemented by the Non-Governmental Organisations (NGOs) at the grassroots.

Influenced by the efforts of Safe Motherhood Initiatives (SMIs) several maternal health projects are initiated by the government. The Health and Population Sector Programme (HPSP) interventions address safe motherhood through: Emergency Obstetric Care (EOC);[2] EsOC; women-friendly hospitals;[3] communication for behaviour change; development and involvement of professional bodies; participation of stakeholders; and the promotion of innovations (Ministry of Health and Family Welfare, 1998b). The EsOC comprises of level of services offered at different health facilities (UNICEF, 1993a). The UHFWC renders first aid EsOC services that include injectable oxytocic (ergometrine), antibiotic and anticonvulsant. At THC and MCWC, basic EsOC services are offered and include first-aid, manual removal of placenta, assisted vaginal delivery and vacuum aspiration. Comprehensive EsOC services including, caesarean section and blood transfusion are offered at District Hospitals and Medical College Hospitals. At present, few MCWCs and THCs are upgraded to render comprehensive EsOC. At village level, the government and NGO paraprofessionals provide antenatal and postnatal care, family planning methods and immunisation. As involvement of TBAs in Safe Motherhood Initiatives did not seem to improve the maternal health, rendering skilled birth assistance through community midwives was suggested in HPSP to ensure safe delivery (Ministry of Health and Family Welfare, 1998a). Thus, the training of community midwives was started to reach maternity care to the community.

In rural Bangladesh, more than 90 percent of births take place at home (Bangladesh Bureau of Statistics, 1997). It is widely accepted that not all births necessitate interventions. Yet, with serious pregnancy complications, indigenous birthing care may not be adequate to save women's lives. Rural women prefer to give birth at home assisted by female relatives or TBAs. My present knowledge on indigenous childbirth practices is built on research conducted in Bangladesh (Afsana & Rashid, 2001; Bhatia, Chakravarty & Faruque, 1980; Blanchet, 1984, 1988, 1991; Goodburn, Gazi & Chowdhury, 1995; Rozario, 1995, 1998, 2002). Their exploration of indigenous birth practices brings to light the issues of cultural knowledge[4] related to pollution and evil spirits that make rural women abide by societal norms and rules. Most researchers debate over the practices of TBAs emphasising on their unhygienic and unskilled practices and associate their low societal status with handling of birth pollution. On the other hand, Goodburn et al. (1995) indicate the usefulness of few indigenous birth practices. Yet, most studies have not considered the potential of indigenous knowledge. None of the studies has addressed the vital role of birthing women and TBAs in birth events. Nor do these studies clarify why women adhere to indigenous birth practices. Even with their simultaneous exposure to the activities of Safe Motherhood Initiatives, it remains ambiguous what exactly makes Bangladeshi, rural women favour indigenously practiced home-birth.

Use of cosmopolitan obstetric care is as yet very low, even when women suffer from complications (Khan, Kanam, Nahar, Nasrin, & Rahman, 2000). Only five percent of 600,000 women with predicted complications are reported to seek hospital care (Ministry of Health and Family Welfare, 1998b). Various studies identify the poor service quality of different hospitals in terms of lack of service facilities, shortage of staff, high cost and inadequate cultural sensitivity (Afsana & Rashid, 2000, 2001; Blanchet, 1988, 1991; Chowdhury, Mahboob & Chowdhury, 2002; Gazi, 1998; Juncker, Khan, & Ahmed, 1996; Juncker & Khanum, 1997; Khan, Kanam, Nahar, Nasrin & Rahman, 2000; World Bank Report, 1999), but, fragmentary pictures of quality are observed in this documentation. Health policy in Bangladesh emphasises the importance of pro-women praxis in health care. Yet, in reality, services for birthing care have been neglected in the existing medical establishment (Bangladesh Fourth Population and Health Project, 1999). In her extensive ethnography of obstetric ward in a district hospital, Leppard (2000) observes that the core values of organisational cultures are developed in hierarchical relationships that give rise to poor quality of care and the social distancing of patients. On the other hand, at societal level, economic reasons, cultural factors and gender relations impede the decision-making process in critical situations of childbirth (Afsana & Rashid, 2000, 2001; Ministry of Health and Family Welfare, 1998b). Notions of purdah[5] also restrict women's use of hospital care in order to maintain their dignity and honour (Afsana & Rashid, 2000). Even then, it is not clearly expressed or documented how rural women's resistance to, or avoidance of using hospital services occurs during childbirth.

Rural women favour indigenous birthing care. However, these processes cannot address birth complications. At present, the reality is that women are dying and suffering (Koblinsky, Campbell & Harlow, 1993; UNICEF, 1993b; NIPORT, 2002). However, maternal deaths and morbidities cannot be attributed to home birth. They occur mainly due to poor socio-economic conditions (Doyal, 1995). Some deaths and morbidities resulting from birth complications can be prevented through modern obstetric interventions (Jordan, 1983; Oakley, 1979), yet actual hospitalisation does not seem to improve maternal health (Tew, 1990). Indigenous knowledge of birth is not encouraged by the Safe Motherhood Initiatives of the State. However, the care women receive in hospital is inadequate (Afsana & Rashid, 2000; Gazi, 1998; Juncker, Khan & Ahmed, 1996; Juncker & Khanum, 1997; World Bank Report, 1999). In order to provide good birthing care, it is vitally important to arrange appropriate care for birth complications and to acknowledge and improve indigenous birth practices in which women can receive effective care as well as confidently participate in their own birth experiences. However, mere endeavour to change birth practices may not result in improvement because the whole system operates in social and political milieux with many individuals and groups. Currently, insufficient information is available about what influences rural, poor women's birth practices. Little is known about what views and thoughts different people hold about it. In response to the dearth of information and the need to improve birthing care, this research aims to explore why and in what ways rural, poor women in Bangladesh adhere to indigenous birth practices and resist to use cosmopolitan obstetric care.

1.2 RESEARCH METHODS AND CONCERNS

I used ethnographic methods, as it is considered essential for this study to obtain deeper understandings of issues (Denzin, 1994) related to childbirth. Jordan (1983) considered this method useful because it gives "the investigator access to the knowing how of birth" (p. 8). However, the new waves of ethnography (Kleinman, 1995) show the way from the objective categories of "tales of the field" (van Mannen, 1988, p. 127) to an interpreted social world where multiple perspectives and voices are heard to achieve deeper understandings of social phenomenon (Denzin, 1997; Guba & Lincoln, 1994). Put differently, the meaning of this phenomenon is explained by the interpretations of the people who live in specific historical, social and cultural context, and face numerous practical challenges and limitations (Altheide & Johnson, 1994). In the context of my research, the use of ethnography provides space for multiphonic interpretations of the observed, the observer, and theory in the social, cultural and political milieux of birth. It is the basis as well as the strength of using the new waves of ethnographic methods in this research.

During ethnographic fieldwork I spent ten months from December 2000 to September 2001 in a village and in the adjacent THC and the Medical College Hospital in Bangladesh. Due to my association with BRAC, a national NGO operating all over rural Bangladesh, I had previously undertaken research in these areas. I chose this village because of my previous acquaintances and familiarity with the local dialect, its close proximity to the hospitals and good road communication. Moreover, I could get an accommodation, located within this village. *Apurbabari* is not an atypical representation of Bangladeshi villages. The THC is situated at the margin of a small town about four kilometres from the village whereas the Medical College Hospital is located in the district town about 23 kilometres away.

In *Apurbabari* village, I selected as key informants women who had experience of both home and hospital birth. I had interactions with them all through the period of fieldwork that significantly deepened my knowledge and experience of indigenous birth. The most enriching experience was the observation of birth events where I not only participated but also listened to the voices of the women as well as the others who participated in the birth. My intention was not to observe essentially the skills of birth attendants, but to understand how everyone, including birthing woman, participated in the event. The interviews were not necessarily formal or even informal question and answer sessions. Rather, they were discussions in which women shared their views. During my stay in the village, I interviewed the TBAs, locally known as *dainis*. Getting to know *dainis*, observing the exercise of their indigenous skills and supportive role and listening to their experiences proved to be a fruitful method of learning about indigenous birth practices. During the course of time I interacted with family members including husbands, parents and parents-in-law, to understand their views and the ways in which they participated in birth events. My interactions with community health workers and field paraprofessionals opened my eyes to their perspectives on birth and their activities in the village. Just as importantly, informal ways of communicating with many other women added to the repository of my knowledge about indigenous birth practices. The more I moved from one place to another, the more I learnt about the existing situation of birth in rural Bangladesh.

Entering hospitals was a real eye-opener on obstetric practices. Viewing the situation through a social researcher's lens was heartbreaking, because I was nurtured in the medical atmosphere in my early academic days. I tried to console myself that perhaps it was different in the good old days but my memories of Kamla's death suggested that little had changed. During the course of my hospital fieldwork, I observed birth events and spoke with the women and their attendants to understand their experiences related to hospital birth. When I sat in wards and labour rooms or walked along corridors, many events happened that I had never envisaged. I observed interactions in medical encounters by accompanying doctors during their visit to patients and I followed nurses when they attended to patients. In the process, I interviewed doctors, nurses, administrators, hospital staff including special *ayahs* and many others who are engaged in constructing birth in hospitals. I took pictures of different events including birth in villages and hospitals, but refrained from clicking cameras during the actual birth process in order not to violate women's privacy.

Ethnographic research produces a huge amount of field text in the form of transcripts and observational field notes (Denzin, 1994). The field notes as well as descriptions of the events that I wrote produced enormous quantities of written observations, and interview notes and transcriptions. My research assistant helped me in recording and transcribing all the interviews I completed in the village. In hospitals, doctors and nurses refused to be recorded on audiotape. Instead, we took notes of their interviews and later reviewed it on our return to residence. I read the research texts again and again and generated themes out of it. The data was eventually presented as narratives with the exposition of verbatim comments in order to enhance the authenticity of the individual voice (Olsen, 1994). While writing the narratives, I presented the experiences of others and the self simultaneously, but carefully kept my position aside and gave prominence to the former. The data I collected were analysed by using a multidimensional framework encompassing culture, gender, socio-economic, political economy and historical perspectives.

The essence of this research lies in documenting the ethnographic details of two contemporary birthing care systems existing in Bangladesh. It is not my contention to compare and contrast these two polarised systems of birth. I present experiences from two systems in order to know the strengths and limitations of each. The significance of this research is that it captures voices and, at the same time, portrays the pictures of events surrounding birth practices that cannot be captured through mere voice. Birthing stories are told and retold by birthing women, *dainis* and other women. It is the women's voice what Foucault (1980a) refers to "subjugated" (p. 81) that brings to light the experiences of the birthing world. Women's absorption in telling their birth stories makes the research participatory. It also contributes to empowering women because they listen to their own voices and reflect on their experiences as a subject worthy of analysis. Furthermore, it addresses the world of obstetric care with the accentuation of medical professionals' voices and practices. The strength of multiple voices is that they are simultaneously homogenous and heterogenous because of the expressions of views from different perspectives. Multiple representations from multiple voices and multiple experiences, including mine, entail many different issues of birth that cannot possibly be explored through the application of singular methods or sources. This methodology is extremely useful to understand deeper issues, but it is limited in its generalisability. Yet, I suggest that the methodology used in this research contributes to the replicability of the approach and techniques in future relevant research.

The issues arising from the study are not only of national significance, but also have international implications, and not only for academic and programmatic interests, but also the interests of women, health care practitioners and feminists. I am not here to critique the worth of one system over the other. What is important to me is to find the strengths and limitations of two contemporaneous practices of birth. The information produced in this research is of immense value in: acknowledging women's indigenous knowledge; highlighting the social, cultural, economic and political influences that affect women's health and health care during birth experience; integrating indigenous birthing care and cosmopolitan obstetrics in a manner that is sensitive to women's needs; and improving the organisation of the existing health care system. As such, the research benefits poor women of rural Bangladesh whose birth experiences are embedded in uncertainty.

1.3 ORGANISATION OF BIRTH EXPERIENCES IN BANGLADESH

This first chapter has provided the backdrop and set the scene and the directions in which the thesis will progress. Chapter two portrays the descriptive features of the research setting where I conducted the fieldwork. The overview of the village and hospitals engages us in comprehending the background of birth practices in Bangladesh.

Chapters three, four and five present the data. In chapter three, I focus on the two birthing systems based on my observations of birth events and the interrelated practices. In the section on indigenous birth practices, I narrate events that happened during the birth experience of one particular woman. With reference to cosmopolitan obstetrics, I chose to describe birth events of two women that occurred in the THC and the Medical College Hospital. The intention of chapter four is to present my observational experiences along with the experiences of women including birthing women, other women and *dainis* who play crucial role in indigenous birth. I describe the role of men, the local healers and the heath practitioners who are directly or indirectly involved in a birth event. In chapter five, I address women's experiences of birth in hospitals, and how the roles of multiple players affect hospital obstetric care. This is strengthened by my experiences of the observation of events. In this chapter, I also present new waves of obstetrics practices by the community health workers and field paraprofessionals in *Apurbabari* village.

Chapter six is concerned with the analysis of findings. To understand the diversity of childbirth, a multidimensional framework encompassing socio-economic, culture, gender, history and political economy is required. Within this broader framework, the significance of this analysis is that it turns the spotlight on indigenous as well as biomedical knowledge with a view to drawing on the components of each that might enhance our understanding of childbirth experiences of rural women in Bangladesh. Chapter seven is the conclusion where I briefly outline the findings, provide answers to the research questions introduced in chapter one, and suggest recommendations that might improve the circumstances of birth for poor, rural, Bangladeshi women.

Notes

[1] I came to know from my grandmother that Majeda was left in front of her house in a small town about 500 kilometres away from Dhaka city. She was a few months old, and was weak and feeble due to malnourishment. My mother and one housemaid took care of her until she became strong. Majeda still introduces her as our sister, but, unfortunately, she was brought up with other maids in our house.

2 EOC includes: Awareness of danger signs (bleeding, severe headache, fits, etc.); Emergency preparedness (knowing when to go where and arranging transport); and Responsive facilities (functional with trained personnel and having necessary drugs and equipment).

3 Women friendly hospital initiative addresses issues of human dignity, women's needs, service availability, views and demands of women and family, services for violence against women, discrimination against women and so on (Ministry of Health and Family Welfare, 1998b).

4 Cultural knowledge is used instead of local beliefs concerning childbirth. The word 'beliefs' has some negative connotations. Beliefs connote uncertainty about 'other' knowledge. For further explanations see B.J. Good in *Medicine, experience and rationality* (1997).

5 One must keep in mind that purdah cannot be universalised. It is not just any seclusion, but a seclusion that has been organised by men of upper classes in favour of women of same classes. Such classes have always been *bhadras* (dominant social forces), primarily geared to the task of keeping intact their identity against the o-bhadras (poor and illiterate). In Islam, the *hijab* or purdah, which literally meant 'curtain,' descended under special circumstances, first to put a barrier not between a man and a woman, but between two men (verse 53 of sura *Ahjab*), and later on to distinguish women aristocrats or 'free women' from women slaves (verse 59 of sura *Ahjab*). In the meantime, the resultant *difference* has been organised and reproduced differently by men in power to the detriment of women. With the 'Islamic invent,' in South Asia, purdah as a system, albeit with certain differences in performance, is shared by the members of all the religious communities of Bangladesh, including those belonging to Buddhist and Christian communities (Ahmed, 1995).

Chapter 2
The Research Scene

This chapter presents the descriptive features of the research setting where I conducted the fieldwork. In the village section, I describe the historical background of the village, geographical features, socio-economic and demographic characteristics, the availability of educational and health facilities, and maternal health-related facts. Subsequently, in describing the THC and the Medical College Hospital, I note the location, structure, facilities, staffing pattern, budgets, hospital utilisation and maternal health statistics. The reason for describing the two health facilities separately, despite some overlap in detail, is that they are different and do have different functions in regard to obstetric care. The overview of the village and the hospitals enables us to comprehend the backdrop of birth practices in Bangladesh.

2.1 THE VILLAGE OF *APURBABARI*

Apurbabari was not the actual name of this village. In Bangla, *Apurba* means beautiful and *bari* means house. I named the village *Apurbabari* because I felt its beauty everywhere. Its original name was named after an influential man who was a Hindu by religion. The reason I raise the religion of the man is that even though all the people living in this village were Muslim, its culture and practice was very much influenced by Hinduism. At this point, I will narrate some features of *Apurbabari*.

Historical Background of *Apurbabari* Culture

In rural Bangladesh, the Bengali, Muslim, rural poor bear the traditions of Islam, Hinduism and Bengali tribal culture as a consequence of different reigns and cultural practices that have been diffused into everyday life over centuries (Maloney, Aziz & Sarker, 1981; Blanchet, 1984; Rozario, 1992). Even then, women, the repositories of cultural knowledge, are little influenced by religion and more by the cultural practices of Bengali traditions (Blanchet, 1984). These cultural practices are observed in childbirth and marriage ceremonies, which are essentially women's domain.

The thana where the village of *Apurbabari* was located was reigned over by a Hindu *Maharaja* (king) during the British period. He became legendary in the locality for his contribution to modern education and to the improvement of water supplies and sewerage systems. The small town of the thana flourished in the late nineteenth and early twentieth century with modern schooling and preventive health care. Yet, the village of *Apurbabari*, which was located only two to three kilometres away from the thana town, has escaped the touch of modernity. Even though, Hindu *Zamindars* (landlords) owned most lands and controlled over local people, the thana was developed during the British period.

In the early centuries, while Brahminical Hinduism became dominant in parts of Bengal, Buddhism and local tribal practices continued to shape the religious culture of common people (Ahmed, 2001). The rigidity of Hindu caste system did not enter into Bengali Muslim Society of East Bengal (Bangladesh), because this area was not of interest to the upper class Hindu Brahminic caste due to its heavy forestation (Eaton, 2001). He (2001) continued to explain that as the river Ganges changed its flow to this part of the Bengal, the land became extremely arable for the cultivation. In the fifteenth and sixteenth centuries, the arability of land drew attention of Mughal regime, which encouraged the petty *mullahs* (Muslim priests), pilgrims returned from Mecca, preachers, charismatic *pirs* (Muslim saints) and local chieftains for the agricultural development of forested hinterland. Although, the Mughals especially Akbar, the Great were very restrictive to conversion of Indigenous people to Islamic faith, this settlement led to construction of mosques or shrines that became the nuclei for the diffusion of Islamic ideals along the agrarian frontier. The seepage occurred over such a long period time that a specific point of conversion of tribal people to Islamic faith was never identified. Rozario (1992) states that it was not the urban oriented Ashrafi Islam, but the Sufi-oriented Islam that pre-dominated the East Bengal. Despite religious and regional distinctiveness, people of East and West Bengal shared a cultural identity due to their common roots in tribalism, Buddhism and Hinduism, which was intensified due to political reform during Pakistani period (Rozario, 1992). However, community as a mode of life predates 'modernity, but communalism as an ideology arises only within modernity (Rozario, 1992).

Village Landscape

The village of *Apurbabari* was located at the Northeast part of Bangladesh. A highway connecting the central and the North-Eastern Bangladesh had gone through the middle of *Apurbabari* dividing it into North and South. However, the village was established a long before the brick road was made. Thus, instead of being North and South, the village continued to be identified with an arbitrary division of East and West as *Pubpara*[1] (East Compound) and *Pashimpara* (West Compound). As I was housed in *Pubpara,* most of my time was spent there. Though I had to move back and forth between both *paras*.

Apurbabari was situated in a flat terrain and surrounded by cultivable lands. At the edge of this village, thana town and three other villages are located. About ten kilometres away from the village were mountainous areas and jungles. These jungles were famous for the trees, which produced good quality woods. What surprised me was the stubbornness of this forest; plants were constantly growing even if trees were uprooted. The village was 20 kilometres from the nearest big river – *Bramhaputra.* Unlike other parts of Bangladesh, it was not affected by flood because of its location in high lands and it's distance from the river. The land was more suitable to growing jute than rice.

The only bazaar was situated at the North end of *Apurbabari*. The highway was running through the heart of the bazaar. On each side of the road were furniture shops, grocery stores, drugstores, tailoring-shops, blacksmith shops, restaurants, tea stalls and *pan* (betel leaf) corners. Moreover, in front of the shops, village men sat in the open place with their gunny sacs or baskets to sell rice and green vegetables. Sheer amounts of fish, chickens and beef were available in the morning. Local buses stopped at the bazaar. Rickshaws and vans were also accessible. The bazaar was primarily a male dominated place. It was the central place where village men socialised and discussed politics, religion and local issues. Besides, most men ate their breakfast and snacks in restaurants and tea stalls. During my fieldwork, I saw one or two old widows buying some goods from bazaar shops. The only brick mosque was located near the bazaar. Men usually attended the Friday prayer there. Women did not go to the mosque. In fact, very few women were able to perform prayers and to read the Koran.

Population Size and Housing Pattern

The villagers claimed that *Apurbabari* was sparsely populated until about forty years ago. Now, the population size is increasing and the cultivable lands are encroached by human dwellers. Recent demographic data indicate that 1154 people resided in about 1.5 square kilometres of land, whereas about 380,000 people live in a 315 square kilometres of land of the total thana (Bangladesh Bureau of Statistics, 2000; Anonymous, 2001a). The ratio of male/female ratio was 0.95 at *Apurbabari* village as opposed to 1:03 at this thana and 1:06 at national level (Bangladesh Bureau of Statistics, 2000; Anonymous, 2001a). As 290 families inhabited the village, at least 400 hundred huts, either tin or straw roofed, were built for shelter. In addition, three small brick houses located in the village belonged to wealthier villagers. People lived in a *bari* (house) with their closely connected relatives. For example, brothers (and occasionally sisters) lived with their children in the same house. Each house had several huts with a small *uthan* (courtyard). In the courtyard, each family owned separate *chulas*[2] where they prepared meals during the dry season. In the rainy season, they cooked either inside their bedroom or in a separate kitchen or in the courtyard by making a small roof over *chula*. The *chula*, in the courtyard, was a place where women socialised while cooking. Unless needed elsewhere, women primarily moved within a *bari* and surrounding areas.

Occupational Pattern

The people living in *Apurbabari* were often economically poor. According to the villagers, most people were previously engaged in preparing mustard oil by hand-operated machine. These people were locally known as *kolu*. Few were engaged in land cultivation and were called *girastha*[3]. As in other parts of Bangladesh, people in this village made fun of *kolu*. They used the metaphoric word '*kolu*' for the less intelligent people who worked relentlessly without making enough money. It suggests that social differences exist between *girastha* and *kolu*. Indeed, during my fieldwork, one wedding was cancelled because the bridegroom came from a *kolu* family. Presently, apart from cultivating lands, the men living in this village had varied occupations including rickshaw puller, bus driver, bus helper, poster painter, plumber, blacksmith, firewood trader, day labourer, small trader, carpenter, barber, jewellery maker, herbalist and healer. Although all the women were homemakers, most were involved in subsistence production. Some women were engaged in different external income earning activities, such as, day labour, small business, tailoring, NGO-run income generating activities, NGO service and so on. Very few families were affluent. Of them, men were engaged in business, and government and NGO services, and women in teaching in government and BRAC primary school.

Literacy and Educational Facilities

The literacy rate (+7 years) was 33.6 percent in the thana, and would presumably be much lower in the village. Most adult men and women were unable to read and write. All the children were enrolled into the government and BRAC's primary education schools. Primary education is free in the government-run primary school, but BRAC charges nominal fees each month. The BRAC School includes not more than 30 students in a five-year schooling programme. The government primary school enrols students far beyond its capacity.[4] Even with the government's sustained impetus for girls' education, very few were seen to continue on to high school. A similar situation was observed among boys. They discontinue schooling, because of lack of study-related support at home and effective guidance at schools.

Water and Sanitation

For drinking and washing purpose, tube-well and the pond water were essentially used. I observed about ten tube-wells installed around the village, some were personally owned and some by the government. The villagers used tube-well water strictly for drinking purposes.[5] There were ten big ponds located in different parts of the village. Pond water was used mainly for washing utensils and clothes, and for bathing. The significance of pond water was that it was mainly intended for purification. The majority did not have an access to safe latrine in their house. They used a bushy place at the edge of the village for defecation. Although, the place of defecation for men and women was separate, unusual situations sometimes created embarrassment. A woman said laughingly, "One evening, I squatted down to defecate, suddenly, I found a man defecating not far from me. I had to run away." For urination, women used a small, closed area built at the backyard of their house, but men urinated everywhere.

Health Care Facilities

The infrastructures of government health facilities extend to the village. The Union Health and Family Welfare Centre (UHFWC) was located about two kilometres, the THC four kilometres and the Medical College Hospital 23 kilometres away from *Apurbabari* village. Within the village along with the government, BRAC organised antenatal and postnatal care, growth monitoring and child immunisation activities for pregnant women and children up to one year of age, with the assistance of field paraprofessionals and community health workers. BRAC also ran supplementary feeding programme for low birth-weight babies under one-year of age. A village home and BRAC schoolroom were used for this purpose. Intrapartum care was mainly home-based, supported by TBAs where most did not receive formal TBA training.

Local health practitioners and healers practised allopathy, homeopathy, ayurvedic medicine, and spiritual healing. Although, most health practitioners were seen to consult patients in private chambers in the evening, they usually visited patients at their house during daytime moving on their bicycles from village to village.

Maternal Health

In *Apurbabari*, the number of women in the reproductive age was 336 and the number of couples was 242. The pregnancy rate was 5.4 percent, which was much higher than the national level of four percent. The attendance of pregnant women at the antenatal care centres was more than 90 percent. In the last five years, no maternal death was reported in this village. During my fieldwork of ten months, among 22 deliveries, 18 had normal deliveries at home and three took place in hospitals, one with pre-eclamptic toxaemia and the other two with prolonged labour. One woman gave birth to premature twins at home who died immediately. Two women reported to have miscarriages.

2.2 THE THANA HEALTH COMPLEX

The Thana Health Complex (THC) was situated at the margin of a thana[6] (sub-district) town. It started as a rural health centre in the mid-nineteen sixties during the Pakistan period. In 1976, it turned into a hospital with 31 beds. Still, in 2001 with increasing population trend, the number of beds remained unchanged. With other health care services, the THC rendered basic essential obstetric care (EsOC).

All the services were offered at no cost. In this section, various aspects of the THC are presented.

Organisational Infrastructure of the THC

In Bangladesh, the Directorate General of Health Services (DGHS) and the Directorate General of Family Planning (DGFP) were two separate wings operating under the Ministry of Health and Family Welfare (MOHFW). The Directorate of Nursing Services (DNS) was a separate unit under which worked nurses in different hierarchies. At thana level, health and family planning worked together under the supervision of a single management. Yet, their budget allocation was issued from two different sources. The Thana Health Administrator (THA) was a medical doctor supervising the whole THC management including field activities.[7] During my fieldwork, a female THA was posted. Under the HPSP implementation, the THC provided three kinds of services – clinical, field and support services. The clinical service, managed by the Residential Medical Officer (RMO), included inpatient, outpatient and emergency care. In this unit worked six medical doctors, nine nurses, two paraprofessionals (medical assistants), one laboratory technician, two pharmacists and one office assistant. The medical officers included one gynaecologist and one junior anaesthetist.

The field service was supervised by one Medical Officer-Maternal and Child Health (MO-MCH). It included an under-five clinic, antenatal and postnatal care, family planning and Expanded Programme on Immunisation (EPI). In this unit of the THC, there were two medical officers, two Family Welfare Visitors (FWVs), one EPI technician and one *ayah* (female ward aide). Many fieldworkers including 65 Family Welfare Assistants (FWAs), 55 Health Assistants (HAs) and eight Assistant Health Inspectors (AHIs) carried out the field activities of MCH programme. The Thana Family Planning Officer (TFPO)[8] provided support services for all the field activities at union and village levels. The staff working in the field service were responsible for carrying out support services.

In the administration office of the THC, ten clerks and one office assistant were posted separately under the Health and the Family Planning wings to carry out accounting and management-related work. Among the hierarchically junior staff, five ward aides (three ward boys and two *ayahs*) and four sweepers (three male and one female) executed support services in hospital premises. In addition, one night guard, one gardener, one driver and one cook were formally posted. Each government employee was entitled to receive one day-leave in a week, and 21 days casual leave and 33 days earned leave in a year.

THC Building and Organisation of Facilities

The hospital was a two-storied building in the middle of two acres of land. The administrative office, outpatient department, emergency room, pathological laboratory, drug-dispensing room and kitchen were located on the ground floor, and wards, labour room and the nurses' room on the first floor of hospital building. The residences for doctors, nurses and other staffs were built inside the compound. A brick wall fenced the whole compound. Outside the hospital gate was the main road where drug stores, corner stores and restaurants were located. Street vendors sold fruit and vegetables there. The distance between the THC and the Medical College Hospital was about 19 kilometres. The ambulance service was available at the THC charging Tk. 240 (US$ 4) to transfer patients to the Medical College Hospital. Road communication was utterly good, and public bus, *tempos*[9] and rickshaws[10] were the principal transportation.

In the hospital building, two wards were located on the first floor, one for women and the other for men. There was no separate maternity or paediatric ward. Child patients were admitted either into female or male ward irrespective of their biological sex. Among 31 hospital beds, 13 beds were seen in the female ward, and extra beds were put according to the needs of the patients. Six beds in female ward were allotted for maternity care, even though, one-thirds of the female patients were pregnancy-related[11].

In the ward, the iron-made beds were set in lines on each side of the room. A foam mattress, rubber-cloth and pillow were placed on this bed. A bed sheet, pillowcase, mosquito net and blanket (in winter) were allotted for each bed. Beside the bed, a small iron locker was kept. A *gamla* (tin bowl) is left under each bed for spitting and throwing rubbish. It was occasionally used as a bedpan. Electric fans were suspended on the ceiling of the roof. The only toilet for women was attached to this ward.

Next to the female ward was the labour room, which were connected by a door. The labour room was lighted by four windows made on the two adjacent brick-walls. A water sink was attached to the side of the second wall near a window. A storeroom was located adjacent to the third wall and a small dressing room behind the fourth wall but remained unused. A long table is placed along the fourth wall. On the table were kept a weighing scale and a drum filled with medicine, gauze and cotton. An oxygen cylinder and a pharyngeal suction machine were put near the table. In the middle of the room, there were two usable labour tables. An old damaged labour table and a baby cot were put at the corner of the room. A ceiling fan was suspended on the top of the roof. A floor lamp placed near the labour table was used in conducting labour. A door leading to the toilet remained closed.

Electricity supply was maintained well. During my fieldwork, water supply was discontinued due to mechanical failure. As the budget for hospital maintenance was issued from different sources and the Department of Public Health Engineering (DPHE) was responsible for this, simple mechanical failure was left non-repaired for months. Four tube wells were installed within the campus for water supply to the hospital. As people fetched water from the conveniently located tubewell, the handles of the other three tube wells were stored in a room for fear of being stolen. Buckets and jugs were used for carrying water. There was no permanent place for garbage disposal. Garbage, thus, was thrown scattered at the back of the hospital building. A steriliser was kept in a small room beside the kitchen. I was not able to observe the steriliser being used during the period of my fieldwork.

Duty Hours of the Staff

The THC had three shifting duty hours in a day. Among the three shifts, the morning shift continued from 8:00 am to 2:00 pm, the evening shift from 2:00 pm to 8:00 pm and the night shift from 8:00 pm to 8:00 am. In the morning shift, all the doctors consulted patients in the outpatient department. Only the RMO attended admitted indoor-patients on ward rounds in the morning and remained on call for 24 hours. In the emergency room, doctors were placed on rotation in different shifts. These doctors were responsible for attending indoor-patients in the evening and at night shifts and on holidays. The nurses were given duty on rotation, and so were *ayahs* and ward boys.

Service Utilisation and Maternal Health

The size of total population in this thana was 387,360 with the number of male being estimated at 197,394 and female at 179,966 (Bangladesh Bureau of Statistics, 2000). The THC documents (Anonymous, 2001b) reported that the numbers of patients attending the outdoor were 78,559 during January-December 2000, and of them, 39,392 were male and 39,167 female. In the same year, a total of 3,045 patients were admitted into the THC. The bed occupancy rate was 112 percent. Of the admitted patients, 1,715 were female admitted with other health problems and 515 are obstetric patients. Among them, 434 women had normal vaginal deliveries, 52 were referred to the hospital and 28 gave stillbirths. One maternal death was documented.

THC Budgetary Allocations

The total annual budget for the THC was Tk. 13,183,224 (US$ 219,720) (Anonymous, 2001b). The DGHS allocated a total of Tk. 7,600,242 and the DGFP a total of Tk. 5,582,982. From the former allocations, Tk. 350,000 (US$ 5,833) was kept for medicine and surgical requisites (MSR). The MSR budget provided Tk. 50,000 to be spent on conveying. The rest of the MSR was used for the following purposes: 75 percent for medicine; 10 percent for instruments; 5 percent for linen; 4 percent for cotton, bandage and gauze; 2 percent for laboratory tests; 2 percent for furniture and others; and 1 percent for oxygen gas.

2.3 THE MEDICAL COLLEGE HOSPITAL

The Medical College Hospital began in 1962 with 500 hospital beds. This hospital was operating along with the old district hospital, which had 146 beds. The old hospital buildings were located at the heart of the city and currently used for infectious disease treatment. The new hospital building were situated at the periphery of the town, which were extended with structures and facilities in the late nineteen sixties. In this hospital, several modern buildings were constructed in a very big compound. The Medical College and the Nursing Training Institution were adjacent to the main hospital buildings. This tertiary, teaching hospital was equipped with full-fledged medical and surgical treatment facilities available in inpatient and outpatient departments. The Obstetric and Gynaecology department offered comprehensive obstetric care. Facilities for laboratory and radiological investigations and blood transfusion were also available. I will present various aspects of the Medical College Hospital, including organisational structures and facilities, in this section.

Hospital Organisational Infrastructure

The Directorate of Health under the direct supervision of the MOHFW managed and controlled the human and financial resources of the hospital. In hospital hierarchy, the position of the Director was the highest. The Director was a medically trained doctor responsible for the total hospital management. In different units of the hospital, doctors and nurses worked. The Professor, Associate Professor and Assistant Professor were teaching staff of the Medical College, but carried out their professional activities in different departments and units of the hospital. There was a Head in each department under whom other professionals worked in different units. During my fieldwork, I found two units in the Obstetric and Gynaecology department where the Head, an Associate Professor was responsible for the administrative procedures of the two units, but was not in-charge of any of them. One Associate Professor and one Assistant Professor were responsible for the overall supervision of each unit. Another Assistant Professor and the Residential Medical Officer, working independently, were assigned to attend patients in some beds in these units. In each unit, the registrar, clinical assistant, junior doctors[12] and intern doctors[13] worked under the supervision of the unit Head. All these staffs with Residential Medical Officer were hospital employee reportable to the Director, Medical College Hospital for official matters.

The Directorate of Nursing supervised the activities of the nurses. In this nursing hierarchy, Nursing Superintendent, Deputy Nursing Superintendent and Nursing Supervisors were posted. In the hospital, all the nurses were reportable to the Nursing Superintendent. In each ward, staff nurses and student nurses worked under the supervision of the Nurse-in-charge who was also a staff nurse. Student nurses reported to the Nursing Institution, but regularly signed hospital attendance registers maintained in Nursing Supervisors' office. The teaching staffs of the Nursing Institution were not directly associated with the hospital administration, but were involved in various activities to improve hospital service quality.

In the government infrastructure, staffs were categorised into various classes: first class; second class; third class; and fourth class. The doctors were the first class employees. Nurses usually belonged to the second and third class, except the Nursing Superintendent and Deputy Nursing Superintendent, who were categorised as the first class officer. The clerical posts were ranked as third class category.

The ward boys, *sarders*,[14] cleaners and *ayahs* were placed in the fourth class and performed the tasks, such as, cleansing, distributing foods, carrying medicine from hospital storeroom and following the orders of the bosses. They were all accountable to the Director of the hospital. In addition, a group of women known as special *ayahs* worked informally in the hospital. They were self-employed and earned livelihood by doing jobs for patients. However, to work in hospital, special *ayahs* had to pay some amount of money, roughly Tk 150 annually to the Fourth-Class Employee Association of the hospital for an identity card.

Organisation of Obstetric Facilities in Hospital

The hospital buildings were four storied. The Obstetric and Gynaecology department was located on the ground floor of two adjacent buildings. The antenatal examination-room, antenatal ward, labour-room, room for eclamptic patients and operating theatre were built in cluster. The two postnatal wards were situated at a distance from the antenatal ward. Each doctor was allocated a single room except intern doctors and few junior doctors. The intern doctors' duty room was located close to the labour room. A common room was also there for the doctors. Tea, TV and newspaper facilities were available in this common room. Some pharmaceutical companies donated a television and a fridge. A seminar room with an adjacent reading room with library facilities was near the antenatal ward and operating theatre. A small room was allocated for the nurses near the labour room. In this room, a telephone-set, equipment (a pot and a stove) for sterilisation, and a storing cabinet for drugs and instruments were kept. Nurses usually sat inside the ward.

In the antenatal examination room, five beds were placed along the walls. The door was screened with curtains. There were six beds in the eclampsia room where in-built oxygen supply and suction facilities were provided. This room, thus, was also used for managing serious obstetric or gynaecology patients. In each of the three wards, that is, one antenatal and two postnatal wards, 24 beds are allocated to patients. Yet, with the increasing patient numbers, additional beds were made on the floor in between two beds. The windows mostly remained closed. In each room, electric fans were hung from the ceiling. There were no particular sitting arrangements for patient's attendants. Each postnatal ward was attached to one toilet. Toilets for antenatal patients were located outside the ward at the corner of the antenatal premises. All the patients from the antenatal ward, antenatal room and labour room used these toilets along with their female attendants.

The labour room was situated at the corner of the obstetric unit. There were five labour beds placed side by side. A long table was put along the wall where the facilities for resuscitating the baby were available. Another table was used for writing patient's notes. Two cupboards were used for storing drugs, cottons, gauzes and bandages. A trolley was set aside for keeping instruments. Two sets of instruments were available in the labour room for performing episiotomy. The instruments were sterilised by boiling in a hot water pot kept in nurse's duty room. A water sink was built in attached to the wall. All the gloves were washed in this sink water and dried on by hanging on a rope line. This room did not have any window. The outer wall of the labour room was made of glass and had an arrangement of exhaust fans, but these fans did not function. A door screened with curtain led to an unventilated wide space inside the hospital building. All these made the labour room stuffy and suffocative.

The operating theatre was situated near the antenatal ward. Surgery was carried out in two operating rooms. Three sets of instruments for caesarean section were available in the operating theatre. The nurse's duty room and postoperative ward were located nearby. The operating rooms and post-operative ward were fully air-conditioned. A few beds were kept in a big space in between the operating rooms and the post-operative ward. Patients and their attendants usually waited there before and during operations. The doctors' changing room, anaesthetists' room and a senior doctor's room were located in this premise. A collapsible gate was made at the entrance of the operating theatre to prohibit free access, and a security guard was always on duty for watching the gate.

The whole hospital compound was fenced by brick wall. Outside the hospital gate was the main road where buses, tempos and rickshaws constantly ran. On each side of the road, drug stores, corner stores, pathological laboratories and restaurants were situated. The residences for doctors, nurses and other staff were built inside the compound, but separated from the main hospital buildings by a brick wall. One tubewell was installed within the main hospital premises, which was the sole source of drinking water. Nine cement-made garbage disposal bins were built in the campus. Rubbish gathered from the hospital was at first kept in garbage bins, and then, put openly in front of one hospital gate. The municipality trucks subsequently collected the hospital waste.

Hospital Shifts

The hospital ran with three shifting hours. The morning shift, in general, continued from 8:00 am to 2:00 pm, the evening shift from 2:00 pm to 8:00 pm and the night shift from 8:00 pm to 8:00 am. The intern doctors, however, carried on the morning shift from 7:00 am to 3:00 pm, the evening shift from 3:00 pm to 10:00 pm and the night shift from 10:00 pm to 7:00 am. For the student nurses, the morning shift lasted from 7:00 am to 2:00 pm, the evening shift from 2:00 pm to 8:00 pm and the night shift from 8:00 pm to 7:00 am. In the morning, the senior doctors attended to the indoor patients, performed surgery in operating theatres and taught students in the hospital or Medical College. The clinical assistants remained on 24-hour call. However, they must perform duty in the morning and usually attended patients at evening and night. The Residential Medical Officer primarily attended to the patients in the outpatient department and simultaneously, attended to inpatients as well. The *ayahs* and ward boys were also placed on rotation through different shifts.

Hospital Utilisation and Maternal Health

The size of total population in this district was 4,439,000 with the number of males estimated at 2,247,000 and females at 2,192,000 (Bangladesh Bureau of Statistics, 2000). The Medical College Hospital document (Anonymous, 2001c) reported that although the number of beds still remained at 646, the total number of patients became more than double each day. The bed occupancy rate was 207%. During July 2000-June 2001 the number of patients attending the Outpatient department was 438,836 and the number of patients admitted to the hospital was 404,732. Among the admitted patients, 9,800 were admitted into the female ward for gynaecological and obstetric problems. Among the 7,287 obstetric patients, 4,098 women had vaginal deliveries, 3,189 caesarean sections and 471 stillbirths and 405 developed eclampsia. The maternal mortality ratio was estimated to be 2,000 per 100,000 live births.

Hospital Budgetary Allocations

The budget was made in accordance with the number of beds. The total annual budget for the Medical College Hospital was Tk. 1,13,399,000

(US$ 1,889,983) (Anonymous, 2001c). There was an annual allocation of Tk. 15,000,000 (US$ 250,000) for medicine and surgical requisites, which was spent on medicine (60%), surgical instruments (15%), linen (6%), cotton, bandage and gauze (6%), oxygen gas (5%), laboratory tests (5%), furniture (2%) and on-costs (1%). Seventy percent of medicine was bought from the government's Essential Drug Company and 30 percent from private companies. The rest of the budget was allocated for human resource management.

2.4 SUMMARY AND CONCLUSION

In this chapter I have presented descriptive features of *Apurbabari* village, the THC and the Medical College Hospital. Like many other villages in Bangladesh, in *Apurbabari*, socio-cultural practices were shaped by the diffusion of local culture and religions. This village was characterised by gradual changes in occupational patterns arising from increasing population size. All women were homemakers and involved in subsistence earning, only some were engaged in earning from outside jobs. The movement of the men was mainly restricted to the village and women were largely confined to the family compound, except those who were involved in income earning. Although education levels were low among the adult population, the current enrolment at primary schools indicated an increasing urge for education. The government health facilities were located within a reasonable distance of *Apurbabari*. In this village, women essentially sought care from *daini* during childbirth. Antenatal care was rendered by BRAC supported by the government field worker.

The THC was located four kilometres away from the village. The service provision at the THC was minimal to address pregnancy complications. On the other hand, the Medical College Hospital, which was located at the district town 23 kilometres away from the village, rendered comprehensive obstetric services. Even with the wide differences in service provision, bed allocation and staffing pattern between the THC and the Medical College Hospital, both the hospitals rendered services to a huge number of patients each day. Yet, this service provision was constrained by financial resources allocated especially for patient care.

The scene that has been set in this chapter comes alive in the next, which describes observational experiences of three birth events. The aim is to understand the lived experience of childbirth practices in *Apurbabari*, the THC and the Medical College Hospital.

Notes

1. *Pubpara* is translated to English as east compound. *Para* is a complex where many households usually belong to kinfolks are located. A village comprises many *paras*.
2. *Chula* is an earthen stove where people cook. People sharing *chula* means that they belong to the same households.
3. *Girastha* is a local term for *grihastha*. In Samsad Bengali-English Dictionary (Biswas, Dasgupta & Sengupta, 1968), *grihastha* is literally translated to (1) a family man; a middle-class man. (2) of or in a house. However, villagers referred it to one who lives on own land and farm.
4. About 100 students start schooling in Class One. By the time, they reach Class V the number of students falls down to 50 (Anonymous, 2001a).
5. Arsenic in tube-well water is the most widespread problem in Bangladesh. The water of one-fourth of the country's 4.3 million tube well is polluted by arsenic. However, in this village, tube wells are declared free of arsenic. The government and NGO have launched programme for arsenic-free water in the affected areas.
6. In the government administrative infrastructure, division, district, thana, union and village are different units in a descending order.
7. The family planning wing used to look after the population control programme including safe motherhood initiatives in the field.
8. As health and family planning is integrated, the TFPO has very little work to do.
9. Four wheeler local automobile
10. Three wheeler human operated cycle
11. Among 1,715 indoor female patients in the THC, 515 are pregnant women in the year 2000.
12. Junior doctors are medical graduate posted in the hospital.
13. An Intern doctor undergoes one-year training in Medical College Hospital after obtaining the final MBBS degree.
14. *Sarder* is a cleaner who supervises the tasks of a small of group of cleaners.

Chapter 3

Two Contemporary Birth Practices: Observational Experiences

At present, rural women seek care from two contemporary birthing systems specifically, indigenous birthing care and cosmopolitan obstetric care. The term indigenous birth has been widely used across the world to signify practices related to homebirth where birthing women along with traditional birth practitioners and other women play a central role. On the other hand, the term cosmopolitan obstetrics is currently being used in childbirth literature to denote modern, hospital based, obstetric care.[1] Here, cosmopolitan obstetrics is used to denote biomedical practices of modern obstetrics, which take place either in the Medical College Hospital, or the Thana Health Complex or home, or village-based antenatal care centres. Even though I have used both the terms – cosmopolitan obstetrics or indigenous birth practices to imply a broad-base, none of the participants in the research are aware of the naming. However, the central issue lies not with the usage of terms, but with what happens to rural, poor women in receiving obstetric care.

In this chapter, I will describe the detailed, narrative features of particular birth events from two contemporary birth practices to exemplify the existing practices and the interactions between different individuals occurring during and after childbirth. To create an understanding of indigenous birthing care, I will present the birth experience of one particular woman from *Apurbabari*. On the other, to describe cosmopolitan obstetrics, I have focused on the birth events of two women, one of which occurred in the THC and the other in the Medical College Hospital. The account of birth events will illuminate how birth is constructed in everyday discourses by the participation of different individuals, and their understandings and interests, and how this construction influences rural poor women's use of birthing care.

3.1 INDIGENOUS BIRTHING CARE

I was passing through *Apurbabari* village. It was a scorching hot day, but beautiful with a blue sky and wonderful clouds. I had to stop. A few women and children were sitting scattered at the backyard of a house. A goat was giving birth. What an extraordinary event was happening! The mother goat was lying down moaning with pain, "*baa, baa* ..." and giving birth to a baby goat with its head coming out first. The mother goat stood up as soon as the baby was born. The baby instantaneously tried hard to stand up along with its mother. The mother goat was licking its body with her tongue. The placenta was hanging from her birth canal. She looked helpless, and perhaps was not appreciating our presence. The goat owner was anxiously waiting for another baby goat to be born with the anticipation of making some cash from selling it. The newly born baby goat was limping around, and to my surprise, made space to put mouth around its mother's nipple. The mother was moving a little restlessly, perhaps having pain in her stomach as the placenta was still hanging. A *daini* in the locality appeared soon and tried to feel another baby inside the goat's abdomen. As she was not able to locate it, the goat owner looked quite disappointed. I had to leave the place shortly. This birthing event happened so naturally that I was mesmerised. Many questions jumbled together in my mind. Is this like an indigenous birthing? What actually happens in human birthing? Why do people consider childbirth as a natural event, though it is socially and politically embraced?

During my medical training from 1983 to 1984, I had great many opportunities to observe and assist in hospital birth. But, I never observed home birth. I still remember several of my cousins gave birth to their first child in our house during my childhood. At that time, one day, I was playing with other kids in our courtyard. The local *daiburi*[2] arrived at house wearing a white *saree*. I knew that something was happening inside the house. All of a sudden, my mother called us in, "Come on children! See the new baby." I found my mother holding a newly born baby on her lap and making wraps with an old cotton *saree* to cover it up. The new mother was lying down on the bed with a smiling but shy face. The *daiburi,* talking to my grandmother, looked very confident. We all surrounded the baby. At that time, a big question was raised in my mind, "How did the baby appear?" I blamed the God for His injustice. I was waiting for a long, but still missed the event when He sent the baby from the sky in a bucket by holding the long rope with one hand. I believed the story for years, because my mother used to explain to us how the baby was born to avoid questions about the whole process of conception and birthing.

I never had the opportunity to observe a home birth until I came to Apurbabari. I waited patiently for this event to happen and never believed that I would really be called in to observe it. A saying exists in the village that circulates from mouth to mouth, "*Joto rao hobe, toto deri hobe baccha houne* (the more people talk about birth event, the more time it requires for giving birth)." Thus, birth events are observed very secretly in *Apurbabari* village. I was apprehensive that if the woman started labour pain at night whether I would not be called in. Luckily, during my stay in *Apurbabari*, I managed to observe several childbirth events and met many women who shared their birthing experiences with me. At this point, I will elaborate my experience with one birth event that occurred in this village.

Birth at Home: Raheemon's Experience

It was in the month of *Ramadan*[3] when I first met Raheemon. She was pregnant - a slender woman with a protruding abdomen. "I will reach full ten months after the next moon, that means, after the month of *Ramadan*," she told me. I estimated her expected date of delivery, which would happen after ten days. At that time, I had just arrived in the village and only introduced myself to the villagers. Within such a short period it was not possible to build up rapport with Raheemon and her family. Besides, in the month of *Ramadan*, no one would have much time to spend with me. I eventually decided not to proceed with Raheemon.

Within two weeks, I came back to *Apurbabari* to begin my fieldwork. At the entrance of *Pubpara* (East Compound) on the main road, Raheemon was standing with her daughter, Morzia near her parents' grocery store, as if waiting to greet us. Her baby was still in her womb. I began my conversation with Raheemon and accompanied her to their house feeling very excited. Many other women also joined us. There was a debate among the women about the expected time of Raheemon's delivery. One woman said, "No, I know her *mashiker shomoy* (menstruation time). She washed her clothes nine and a half months ago. The baby will not be born before the next moon appears. So, 15 more days to wait." Raheemon looked very irritated and annoyed as the women were delaying her due date of delivery. Perhaps she wanted to get rid of her huge bulky abdomen soon.

Raheemon was about 22 years old living with her parents. Her husband lived in the district town about 20 kilometres away from the village. He was considered 'abnormal' in this village, as his behaviour and personality seemed widely divergent. He worked in a baking factory and earned very little to support the family. Raheemon took credit from an NGO and invested money in her parent's grocery store. She shared the same *chula* with her parents and largely took care of household chores. She was not seen running here and there, instead she was busy preparing food and doing other household chores steadily. In the course of three weeks, I was able to develop an agreeable, friendly relationship with Raheemon and her family. I used to converse in between her chores in the morning, at noon, in the afternoon and in the evening. She shared the tale of her first birth experience, and gave me ideas as to what norms and rules were being followed before, during and after birth events, women's participation in birth experiences, and the role of *daini*s in birth events. During our discussion, I came to know about her grandmother, Taljan Bibi, who was an eminent *daini* in the locality. I created space and time to get acquainted and converse with Taljan Bibi who would be assisting in Raheemon's birth event. I spent most of my time in their house building rapport and interviewing Raheemon, her grandmother, mother and father and the neighbours.

At the time of her first pregnancy, Raheemon lived in her parents-in-law's house, which was located in the district town. She had to observe the norms and rules of pregnancy in spite of living in a town. She was not allowed to go out alone at noon or in the evening, or on Tuesday or Saturday. Raheemon did not follow many restrictions regarding food. She said, "I don't believe in food taboos. I used to eat all foods before my daughter was born." Her baby girl was born at home. Her mother-in-law, who was also known as a *daini* in the locality, assisted in birthing. Raheemon was saying:

> I was having *kini kini bedna* (little pain) for two to three days. I didn't tell anyone, as you know, the period of labour pain prolongs if more people come to know about it. But my sister-in-law understood that I was developing *baccha houner bedna* (labour pain). I was doing my normal household chores, like cooking and cleaning. In the

evening, after dinner, I really started pain in my belly. My mother-in-law came in and touched my belly and tried to feel the baby. She said, "It will take bit longer." I was a bit scared, but one has to keep *moner shahosh* (mental strength) during childbirth. The baby was born normally very early in the morning without any problem. My mother came in the following day. She also knows how to deliver the baby, but didn't come forward as my mother-in-law decided to assist in the birth. After all, it is *porer ghorer baccha* (the baby belongs to the other family). What will my mother and I say if some mishaps happen to the baby during delivery? My mother did all the tasks in *chodighar* (seclusion room).

In that afternoon, while writing field notes in my room, I heard voices outside. Someone was calling me, "*Apa, Apa* (sister, sister), please open the door." Begom, Raheemon's sister stood in front of the door along with other girls. Begom said excitedly, "My sister is requesting you to visit our house." I said, "Why?" "I don't know, please come with us." We all went together. Raheemon was waiting for us in their shared bedroom. An eating-place was set on the bed with nicely decorated napkins. I saw earlier at noon Raheemon cooking some special foods. It was then 3:30 pm. Raheemon said, "*Apa*, I always feel bad. You come and sit in our house everyday, but we do not offer you anything to eat. I am not very well now and couldn't prepare many items. Please eat with us whatever I cooked." I know Bengali hospitality, but did not expect it from an economically insolvent family. I was ashamed of myself because I used to visit them with a purpose, but she was genuine in showing respect and hospitality. How do I return such genuine friendship and hospitality? On my return, I told my research assistant, "The day before my son was born, I had a very big dinner. I feel that Raheemon will be giving birth tomorrow."

It was a dark, cold night. My research assistant and I were in deep sleep. Suddenly, I heard whispering voices near the windowpane, "*Apa, Apa*." Both of us jumped out, opened the door and found a group of women standing there. One of them said, "Raheemon has started labour pain." We immediately got dressed up and moved to Raheemon's house. My dream was coming true. I felt excited, but was little panicked because I never had the experience of watching with my own eyes a *daini*-assisted home birthing.

We arrived at Raheemon's house. The neighbourhood was quiet and sleeping. Raheemon was moaning with pain. She wore an old petticoat and blouse covering her upper body with a shawl. She was standing at

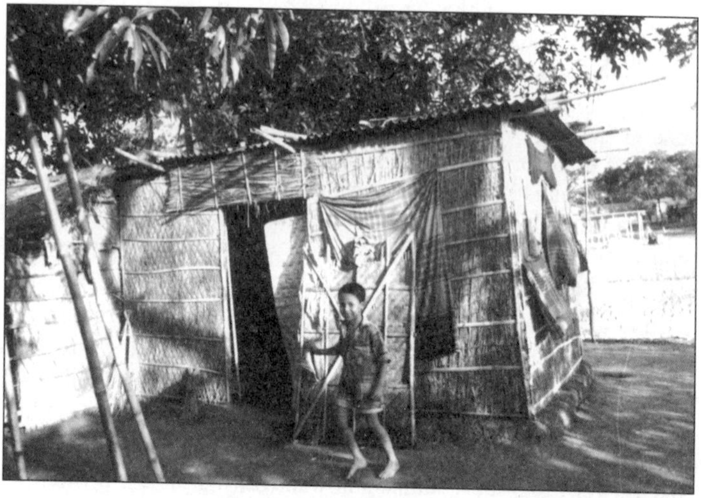

Photo 1: A village hut

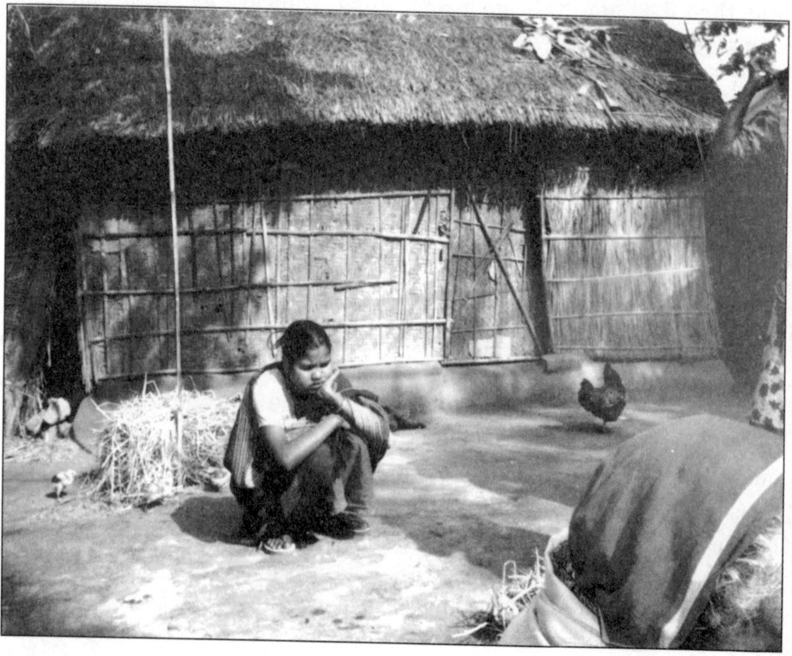

Photo 2: Raheemon sat in the courtyard in front of Taljan's hut

the corner of the veranda, an elongated open space attached to the front side of their bedroom. At the other corner of the veranda, goats were sleeping in a fenced area. In the middle, a fireplace was set with sticks and straws where Taljan and two other women sat to warm them up. I met Ambika, Raheemon's mother who came out of their bedroom. Raheemon's father and daughter were sleeping inside. Raheemon started to walk along the veranda and courtyard. She was shivering with cold and asking for the God's blessings. Ambika brought a jute-sack to make a floor bed for Raheemon and a handmade, cotton quilt to cover her up. I could sense that Taljan did not like our appearance on the scene. Afterwards, she told me, "I was hesitant when they called you. You know, the birthing process becomes longer as more people come to know about it, and it surely happened to Raheemon."

Women sitting around the fire were sharing their birthing experiences. They talked about the issues of courage, fear, death, and pain related to childbirth. One woman said, "It is crucial to have mental and physical strength during childbirth. If you don't have it, you can't give birth." Another woman was saying, "It is right. But, if *kol-bekol* (problem) happens, you can't give birth normally even if you have both mental and physical strength." In this context, Taljan commented,

> Yes, I agree. But, nowadays, it has become a fashion to go to the hospital for birthing. That child could be born at home, but if labour pain is prolonged, the family takes their wife or daughter immediately to the hospital.

Another woman stated,

> In our time, I was working and didn't let anyone know about my labour pain. I could feel my baby would be coming out soon. I went into my bedroom, sat on the floor, held the bamboo pole, pushed two or three times and the baby came out. Then, I called my mother-in-law to cut the cord. It's the birthing woman who is responsible for giving birth to a baby. I don't like someone touching me. I know some bad *daini* who make the area swollen and sore. The good ones never touch, they usually wait and occasionally intervene.

Taljan again said, "When my last child was born, I was working, processing rice. I was not able to put the third pot of rice on the *chula*. I had to rush. The baby was born, but it was dead." Women talked about death without any hesitation when a new birth was expected to happen. Ambika noted, "I felt that my baby was not moving anymore. I told my sisters-in-law. They encouraged me to have patience. After a day or two, a dead baby was born." All the women participating in the discussion had a history of at least one baby who had died either before or right after birth.

Raheemon was still lying on the jute sack quietly. Taljan said, "If she had much pain, she would not be able to lie down so quietly. She doesn't seem to have much pain, now." Raheemon responded sharply with yelling voice, "Shut up, old lady. I am dying of pain and you are saying, I don't have pain." All the women started to laugh at her. One woman described experience of her own labour pain. She noted, "I felt so much pain during my labour. I still fear." The other woman said, "I don't feel much pain during labour, but my after pain is very severe." In this regard, Taljan commented, "It is called *adla bedna*. If a woman having *adla bedna* touches the birthing mother, she also develops it. My daughter got it from me and passed it on to Raheemon." Raheemon was moaning and bending her body in pain. Ambika told her, "Don't bend your body." Raheemon stood up and went across the courtyard behind the neighbour's hut to evacuate her bladder. She tried to squat by bending her body forwards and touching the ground with the upper limbs, and began to urinate slowly. She looked a little exhausted. I asked her, "How do you feel now?" She said, "Alright!"

I sat with the women also to get warmth from the fire. Women began to talk about fear of death. One woman stated, "Every woman fears death. Though becoming pregnant and giving live birth are happy moments." Another one said, "Whenever I think of being pregnant, fear encroaches on my heart. Pregnancy is so common in our life, yet still we fear." Sharoma added,

> Women follow many social rules and norms to have a safe birth. I got very worried when I became pregnant. I saw my aunt die of bleeding during childbirth. I saw my sister's two babies pass away after being born alive. We don't know for what reasons mishaps happen during childbirth. We face so many uncertainties that we even ask for forgiveness during delivery.

"Many lives of mothers and babies are sacrificed in childbirth. Perhaps that creates fear in the mind of women and their families," commented Ambika.

The sky was becoming clear. Daylight was approaching. *Pubpara* was waking from sleep. The warmth and brightness of fire were diminishing. Taljan and the other women got up and started their chores. Ambika let the goats off from the fenced place by the veranda and took them away to the grazing land. A birthing place was built up at the corner of the veranda walled by a bamboo partition. Raheemon was lying down there. The neighbours came in, and peeped inside. Some also advised her. One woman said, "Raheemon, why do you lie down? It's not good for your birthing. Stand up and walk. Shake your legs and hands." Raheemon stood up and shook her both legs and hands several times. Then, she started to stroll down. She repeated shaking her legs and upper limbs. After a while, she sat down to take a rest. Everyone in the house ate breakfast prepared from last night's leftover meal. Raheemon was also given *korkora bhat*[4] to eat. She ate some, and soon vomited out. She again lay down with her little daughter on the jute sack covering their bodies with warm quilts.

While women sat around the fire, they were also joking with each other. Most jokes were about their own birth experiences. Kamila was sharing her stories by making bodily gestures, "I had terrible pain. I was jumping up and down. My mother held me tight. Even then, I did not stop." Women laughed. Sharoma shared her experience,

It was not my full month. I did not realise that I developed labour pain. I felt stomach cramps and rushed to the backyard. Suddenly, I heard a baby's cry. I started to scream calling my mother, "*Ma, come and see*." The baby was just lying on the ground. My mother came at once. Everyone started to run all over the place. I felt very stupid. It's not even my first baby. I always tried to be smart before everyone. Now, everyone was smiling at me as if they were saying – stupid woman, didn't you understand labour pain?

Ambika described how she learnt *daini*'s work starting first with a goat delivery. Anwara mentioned that she saw a male *dai* in her relative's birth event. Everyone smiled at each other. Chatting was going on all around.

Abdul Jabber, Raheemon's father, came out of their bedroom with his eyes downward. He slipped away from the house. I found out that none of the men were inside the household premises. One woman said, 'Now, men will go out for work. When a birth event takes place, men do not stay inside the house. It is not only a matter of *sharam*[5] for women but also for men." I have observed the same event in another house where birth occurred at very late night. All the men spent the night in a neighbour's courtyard, but they were called in to discuss a matter if felt necessary. Whatever was possible for men to do, they agreeably did a range of tasks from buying blades to collecting matchsticks, lighting lamps and fetching *dainis* from their house. In a different situation, where I referred a woman to the THC, all the men in this house and a few male neighbours sat together to discuss about how to travel, where to get money, and who would be accompanying.

It was seven in the morning. Ambika stood before Raheemon and put some mustard oil on her *mathar chandi* – top of the head. She pulled a few of her hair locks along the front of the chest towards her belly button and drew some mustard oil from her head along the hair locks to her abdomen. Then, she massaged this oil over Raheemon's abdomen and shook her waist a few times. Raheemon sat on the floor and asked her mother to massage her thigh and upper limbs. Ambika followed her daughter's instructions and pressed limbs.

The neighbours and relatives came now and then. One woman commented, "It's not good to have a baby during daytime. People disturb a lot." An old lady came in and told Ambika to offer Raheemon a plate of warm rice. Meanwhile, Ambika cooked rice and fed Raheemon warm rice mixed with green chillies and mustard oil with her own hand. She was moaning with pain but ate rice very quickly. It was about ten in the morning. Ambika and Taljan seemed impatient. They sent Begom to obtain pain enhancing plant roots from a local healer named Halem *Fakir*. After sometime, Begom came back unsuccessfully. Ambika looked anxious running to-and-fro from courtyard to veranda.

Raheemon seemed controlled and occasionally asked her mother to massage her limbs. She stood up, and all of a sudden, water was seen trickling down her legs. Taljan came nearer. Raheemon's pain was increasing. She was calling the God's name. Raheemon took a reclining position. Ambika and Marium sat behind her with their hair laid loose. Taljan sat near Raheemon's feet. She tried to examine the birth canal with the left index finger after dipping in mustard oil, "*Shoriler mukh khulse* (the mouth of uterus is open)." Then, she sat facing the mouth of the birth canal by spreading Raheemon's both legs. All the women sitting there had their hair laid open. My hair was short, so I was not asked to do anything with my hair. I sat beside Raheemon's right leg. Raheemon started to push down and said, "Please grandma, put your big toe on my arsehole." Taljan sat against the bamboo wall and guarded the perineum by placing her big toes on the anus. Raheemon was bearing down. The baby's head was seen through the opening of the birth canal. Raheemon pushed down hard four to five times. Taljan wrapped her left hand with a piece of cotton fabric to get the baby out. She said, "It's very slippery." The baby came out encased in an almost intact amniotic sac. It was placed uncovered on the jute sack near its mother's leg. Now, the women became busy with delivering the placenta. One of them pushed Raheemon's long hair inside her mouth to stimulate vomiting. She wanted to vomit several times. Taljan was holding the cord with her left hand and the placenta came out spontaneously.

The baby was still lying on the jute sack inside the bag. Taljan was surprised, "I have never seen a baby in a bag. It is all Allah's wish." She tore the bag with fingers and pulled blood from the placenta towards the baby by squeezing the cord. Taljan was looking for a blade and thread. Everyone was running all over the place to find a blade. Then, Begom handed it to Taljan, who tied the cord with dry threads and severed it with a new blade. I was told that the blade was boiled in hot water. However, I saw that water was left on a *chula* for hours but it was not boiled, and the blade was just washed in warm water. Taljan put some blood into the baby's eyes from the incised end of the cord and said, "This boy will not be a *luccha* (ill-character). He will have some *sharam* (shyness and modesty) in his eyes and will not look at women by keeping eyes open and straight."

The baby was taken out to the courtyard for a wash. The mother was left alone sitting still on the jute sack. She was bleeding and moaning with pain. The neighbouring women gathered on the courtyard with a group of children. The baby was given a bath with soap and stove warmed pond water. It was wrapped in dry old clothes and taken to the sun. Begom was sitting on the ground placing the baby on her lap. She rubbed mustard oil on its body, and wiped his mouth and nostrils with it. Meanwhile, Ambika managed to bring cow's milk from a neighbour's house and warmed it up. Begom put warm cow's milk mixed with sugar into the baby's mouth. The neighbours were watching all the events and giving instructions, but nobody came forward for assistance in fear of getting polluted. Ambika and Taljan helped Raheemon to take a bath. Ambika poured warm water on Raheemon's body. Raheemon washed her body with soap and water, and changed her dress. She was still bleeding, but did not cover her bleeding areas with clothes. A jute sack was placed over a hot brick in the courtyard for Raheemon. She sat on this jute sack enjoying the warm sunlight. Now, the baby was placed on her lap.

Abdul Jaber, Raheemon's father came in with another man. In Islam, *azan* is said if a boy is born. The man said *azan* because the newly born baby was a boy. Abdul Jaber looked very happy and cheerful. Ambika said, "A grandson is born. Will he not be happy?" In the meantime, Abdul Jaber went to the local drugstore to buy some medicine for his daughter's after-pain. He gave some tablets to his wife and said, "This is for Raheemon. It will reduce her pain." Ambika told me, "I didn't ask him to buy any medicine. He did it on his own."

Raheemon was waiting outside in the courtyard. The room was still not ready. Taljan removed the soiled torn clothes and placenta, and buried them at the backyard. Ambika started mopping up the veranda floor and the adjacent courtyard and smeared it with clay-water. The quilts and jute sack were taken to the pond for washing. Raheemon seemed very hungry. She was the one who did the kitchen chores. As Ambika was busy with other chores, a meal was not yet prepared. The common scenario in a village is that the neighbours usually help in cooking meals, chopping vegetables and lighting and keeping on fire or *chula*. Today, neighbours came to see the baby, but not a single one showed keenness to give a hand in their household work.

A bed was set for Raheemon inside their only bedroom. Straws and jute sacks were placed on the floor covered with cotton quilts. Raheemon entered into the room to observe her period of confinement that would continue till the seventh day of childbirth. A fire was lit with a small tree stump and put near the floor-bed. Ambika said,

> In a *chodighar*[6], one always needs fire. You can warm up milk. You can make your finger warm and press it around the baby's belly button. You can make *kajol*[7] and put a black *futa* (round mark) on baby's forehead. Fire also keeps the *hydor* (evil spirit) away from the baby and the mother.

The room seemed very stuffy. I was worried about the consequences of smoke on the baby's respiratory tract. Hashi, a neighbour said "Nothing will happen to them. In fact, it's good for health." The baby was lying down on the floor bed wrapped up in clothes. A bundle of items wrapped up with a piece of fishing net was kept near the baby's head. This bundle included *khodar gorur haar*[8] (cow bone), iron knife, *hachon* (bamboo broomsticks) and a branch of *nishinda* (local tree leaves. A matchbox was also kept. When Raheemon went out, she carried *nishinda* leaves, broomsticks and the matchbox to keep away *batash* (evil wind) and *hydor* (evil spirits). Before entering into the room or touching the baby, her body and breast was touched with leaves and sticks to remove spirits. A brick was also kept near her bed and made warm on the fire to put hot compress on her perineal area. Raheemon was not wearing any clothes for vaginal bleeding. She wore a petticoat and frequently changed it. She sat on the hot brick covered with jute sack to warm her feeble body.

Raheemon was not given anything to eat till Ambika cooked an afternoon meal. She ate rice with *aloo chana* (mashed potatoes) mixed with green chillies and mustard oil. Till the seventh day, she ate only rice and mashed vegetables and did not even touch lentils. As Raheemon said,

> I did not follow any food restrictions during my pregnancy period. But, now I have to follow it to keep *hydor* away from my baby. I can't eat fish and meat products. I can't do anything that will harm my baby.

Another woman standing there said, "In our family, we eat fish, but not the scaly ones. *Hydor* comes with scaly fish." In most families, fish and meat products were restricted for birthing women.

In the evening, I found Raheemon and her baby sleeping together. The baby was wrapped up in quilts, sleeping like a big cotton ball near his mother's chest. His forehead was marked with a black round mark and lower eyelid coated with eyeliner made from *kajol*. The fire was blazing with short flames. After sunset Raheemon was not allowed to go out to empty her bladder and bowel. A long piece of banana bark was placed at the corner of the room as a urine pan. She urinated at one end of the bark, and urine was drained out through the other end placed at a floor hole. Raheemon did not evacuate her bowels at night, but usually newspaper was used for this purpose. Ambika spent the night in the same room, but Abdul Jaber slept at their store for forty days. Morzia stopped to demand her mother's breast milk as soon as her brother was born. The newly born baby was fed breast milk and cow's milk as well.

Till the seventh day, Raheemon observed the same routine. Each morning the baby was put in the sun after his body was massaged with mustard oil. The bundle of leaves, cow bone and a matchbox were always kept near the baby's bed. Raheemon gave him a bath with stove-warm pond water. One day, I found Raheemon very upset. No one was preparing warm water for her baby's bath. During the period of confinement, Raheemon was not allowed to touch the *chula*. She took a neighbour's assistance in fetching water from the pond, lighting the *chula* and warming up water. Then, she bathed her baby with this warm water. Raheemon was sobbing, "No one is helping me. My mother looks after the store, cooks, cleans and washes, but Begom doesn't want to do anything." Begom furiously said, "Of course, I do. I look after Morzia, make breakfast, sweep the house and do lots of things. You can't get upset. It may happen in a busy house." The baby was placed in the sun again. Raheemon finished her bathing at the back of the neighbour's hut. After taking bath, she ate freshly cooked warm rice and mashed vegetables. Raheemon and the baby went inside the room before noon.

Lights were kept lit for the whole night in the baby's room for the first six nights. To keep the *hydor* away from the baby, either Raheemon or Ambika stayed awake. Raheemon sat down every now and then holding the baby in her lap and giving warm compress around the belly button by warming her thumb. If Raheemon fell asleep, Ambika woke her up. Raheemon or Ambika lay down holding the baby close to their chest. There is a saying in the village, "The baby sleeping at mother's back does not survive long." Raheemon's son slept well getting the body warmth from his mother and grandmother.

On the seventh day, a ceremony named as *choditula*[9] was observed. I arrived early in the morning at Raheemon's house. The barber arrived around ten in the morning to shave the baby's head and to cut his finger and toe nails. A *kula*[10] was garnished with betel leaf and nut, tuft of paddy, some grasses, lighted *matir prodip*[11], onion turmeric and others. Taljan put the baby on her knees holding him with both hands. The barber shaved the baby's head with a steel blade. Taljan told the barber, "You are supposed to use a *khur*[12]. Why are you using a blade? Do you think it will remove *napak* (pollution)?" The barber said mockingly, "*Nani* (grandma), where will you get a *khur* nowadays? This blade will serve the same purpose." However, Taljan insisted on the importance of using *khur*. Meanwhile, I observed Raheemon shortening her own nails. Taljan asked the barber to cut down baby's nails, but he refused. Taljan did not like it. She said "What will barber do then? Only shaving head?" After shaving was done, the barber was offered an amount of Tk. 10, half a kilogram of rice, mustard oil, onion, salt and turmeric. However, the barber declined to accept it, as the offering was lower than the typical one given in such ceremonies. Taljan again bargained. She said, "We will give you the rest on the 14th day when you will come to shave baby's head again." The barber looked slightly annoyed and left the house immediately. The neighbouring women told Taljan not to bargain with a barber, "No one should deprive the barber of his due fees. It is not good for the well-being of the baby." Raheemon was also annoyed with her grandmother. I assumed that the barber left angrily, but later on discovered that he went out for taking bath in the pond. The barber was given the standard fees.

The bath of a birthing woman was ceremonious. As soon as the baby's bath was over, Raheemon went to the pond. She took a bath in the pond going down under water three times to remove pollution. She scrubbed her body and cleansed thoroughly. She washed her *saree* and other clothes while taking bath. After drying herself, Raheemon wore a clean *saree* and hung her clothes on the rope line in the courtyard. Now, she became free of pollution and was allowed to touch the *chula*. Raheemon warmed milk and fed her son. Then, she sat near the *chula* to help her mother.

The rituals of cleansing were initiated earlier in the morning. Raheemon's bed was removed from the floor. Begom cleaned the whole house by smearing the floor of the room and veranda and courtyard with mud and cow-dung and washed household utensils in pond water. Ambika washed all the clothes, which came in contact with Raheemon and her son. The clothes were boiled with soap and pond water, and washed in the pond. The pillows and mattresses were dried in the sun. Raheemon's bed was now made on the *chowki*[13] where she usually slept. From now on, Morzia would be able to sleep with her mother. Even though, Raheemon was allowed to do all the household chores, in general, birthing women perform light work till 40 days of childbirth. Moreover, full purification was not achieved until 40 days when she would perform prayers.

3.2 ARRIVAL OF COSMOPOLITAN OBSTETRICS

I talked to a group of women to identify when exactly women from *Apurbabari* village started to use cosmopolitan obstetric services. I coincidentally met Zahirun Begum while interviewing her sister-in-law, one of my key informants. My conversations discovered that Zahirun sought hospital obstetric care in the late nineteen sixties. At that time, very few were aware of this kind of care. Zahirun was taken to the same Medical College Hospital where I did my fieldwork, to get treatment for antepartum eclampsia. She had been unconscious for two days. Her baby was born in the hospital. She did even not know what medications were given to her. Later, the family learnt that Zahirun was given wrong medications. Hospital doctors and nurses were frightened of their therapeutic negligence. When Zahirun left the hospital, one senior doctor gave her Tk. 100 in consideration of her poor economic situation. She commented, "Days have changed. Can you think of giving money to a patient now? Doctors now suck money from the patient till the last penny is gone." Even though, Zahirun was not positive or encouraging about hospital birth, she bore good memories of the kind and caring attitudes of few doctors and nurses. The experience from the late sixties gives us some impressions on how woman felt about hospital obstetric care. The recent observations of birth events will illuminate about how rural, poor women experience birth in hospitals.

Birth in the THC: Rahena's Experience

More than three decades later, I was sitting in the nurses' room at the THC. It was late morning, and the day was gloomy with the sky covered with grey clouds. Sometimes, the sun was trying to peep through the holes of grey clouds. The Health Complex was busy as usual. Men, women and children came in and went off. Visitors were sitting on the patients' beds and on the benches, eating foods, chatting with each other and also spitting on the floor. The vendors were selling *jhal muri* (chilli puffed rice), biscuits, *and paan* (betel leaf) and cigarettes. As facilities for treating serious illness are not available at the THC, most patients I found were not seriously ill. Thus, the atmosphere did not seem like a 'real' hospital. The female cleaner was sweeping up the floor with broomsticks. One *ayah* was sitting in the nurses' room. The male cleaners and ward boys were moving here and there - busy for no apparent reason. The nurses were roaming around in a relaxed manner. The RMO was expected to pay a visit soon. It is important to note that during my fieldwork I did not see other doctors attending indoor patients in wards during morning round.

While I was talking to the nurses in their room, suddenly, a group of men and women appeared with a young woman who was moaning with labour pains. They all disappeared into the female ward. A young man entered into the nurses' room with some paper sheets. One nurse asked him about the birthing woman's condition. I decided to visit the woman. On my way to the labour room, I crossed the veranda, where four to five men accompanying the birthing woman were waiting anxiously. I entered into the female ward, which smelled fetid and looked dirty. Flies were seen everywhere sitting on patients' beds, and on the floor. Fetid odor was emitting from the attached toilet. For more than five to six months, the water supply had been discontinued due to mechanical problems. Since then it was left without repair. Presently, water was fetched from the tube well located on the campus a little away from the main hospital building. The water supply problem gave the cleaners an excuse not to cleanse the hospital building regularly.

I quickly moved to the labour room. The curtained door remained closed. I opened the door and carefully removed the curtain, as the nurses regularly used it for wiping their hands. The labour room was crowded with women came with the birthing woman. One woman lying on a labour table had just given birth and was still attached to her saline drip. The newly admitted woman was approaching the other table. The room was messy and stunk with urine. Windows were left open and screened with curtains. They were also used for wiping hands. The floor, in some places, was stained with blood. Cotton-balls and pieces of bandage were scattered on the floor. In the attached storeroom, I saw clean bed sheets and pillows, which were kept locked and unused in fear of being stolen and soiled. Of the three labour tables, two were in use. At the corner of the room, a baby-cot was left in which few ragged mattresses and pillows were dumped. A table at the corner was messy and sticky with dirt.

Rahena, the birthing woman, was trying to climb up onto the labour table with the help of her attendants. She was about 19 years old and was pregnant for the first time. Two nurses came in with the *ayah*. The nurses asked the *ayah* to fetch water from the tube well, but she did not pay attention to their requests. One of the nurses again asked the *ayah*, who then managed to send Rahena's relatives to fetch water. One of the nurses picked up a glove, which was hung along with other washed gloves on a jute rope line. She asked Rahena to remove garments to have a better exposure of her vaginal area. The first nurse did a vaginal examination and asked the other nurse to prepare a medicine list for Rahena. The second nurse looked for papers to order a list of medicines. These medicines were not available in the THC. She passed on the list to a female relative, who happened to be a *daini*. Rahena was in pain. The first nurse said, "The cervix is almost dilated, but the pain is not very strong. Please send someone to bring medicine quickly." The female relative went out. The second nurse removed the saline set from the other birthing women, and inserted the same needle into Rahena's vein.

Within 15 minutes, the prescribed medicine arrived along with a bottle of coconut oil. I came to know from a village *daini* about the use of coconut oil as vaginal lubricants in hospital, but did not fully believe her. To my surprise, the first nurse poured coconut oil on her gloved hands and over the vaginal orifice and inserted her hand inside vagina. She was trying forcefully to dilate the mouth of cervix and stretch the vaginal wall with her fingers. She said, "Look, how the *daini* made the swelling of vaginal orifice." I looked but did not find any swollen area. The first nurse asked for some clothes to guard the perineum. One female relative brought out some ragged pieces of clothes from a bag and handed in to the nurses. The second nurse injected medicine in the saline bag. She stood on the right side of Rahena and tried to stretch the anterior wall of vagina with her gloved hand. After a while, I found a tear on the vaginal orifice near the labia minora. I asked, "How did it happen?" "It just happened now. We will stitch it." The way she was handling the birth passage, I myself felt pain inside my vagina. Rahena was whispering, "Please help me God. I can't bear it anymore." The nurse became irritated and scolded Rahena harshly for not pushing hard. Rahena tried hard to push down but in silence. The first nurse was continually dilating the passage. The second one held her right leg and the *ayah* her left leg. The first nurse asked for more coconut oil. Rahena wanted to straighten her legs, but was not allowed to. Her back was hurting, but none of her relatives dared to touch her back.

The two nurses struggled with Rahena's birth passage. After struggling for sometime, the baby's head was seen. The female relatives and the accompanying *daini* started reciting Koranic verses. The situation became depressing and frightful. The first nurse gave episiotomy incision on the perineal area with a non-sterilised scissor. The baby was brought out forcefully with some physical efforts. It was slightly cyanosed and did not cry. The female relatives looked anxious. After cutting the cord, the baby was given to the *ayah*. The *ayah* said irritatingly to the female relatives, "Couldn't you pass me some ragged clothes?" One of them gave her clothes and waited near the baby. The *ayah* started to resuscitate the baby by giving oxygen and suction in mouth and throat. She injected sodium-bi-carbonate into the cord. Suddenly, the Residential Medical Officer (RMO) came into the labour room side while doing morning round. It was quite unusual in this THC for a male doctor to appear in the labour room. He looked a bit

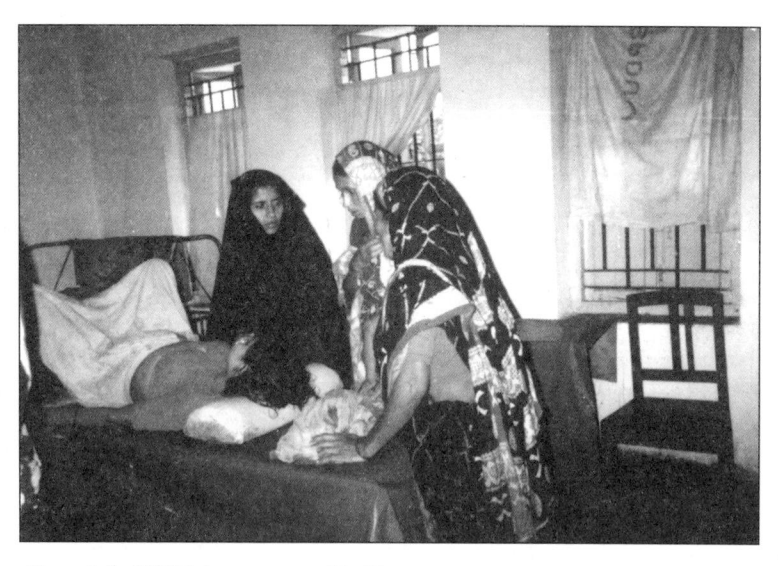

Photo 3: In THC labour room, a birthing woman was surrounded by relatives

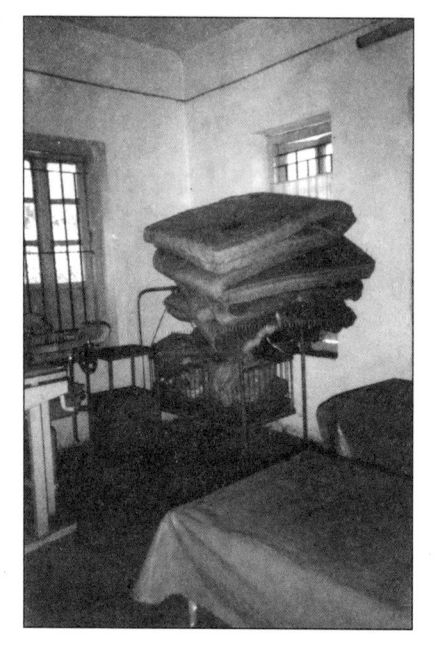

Photo 4: The THC labour room

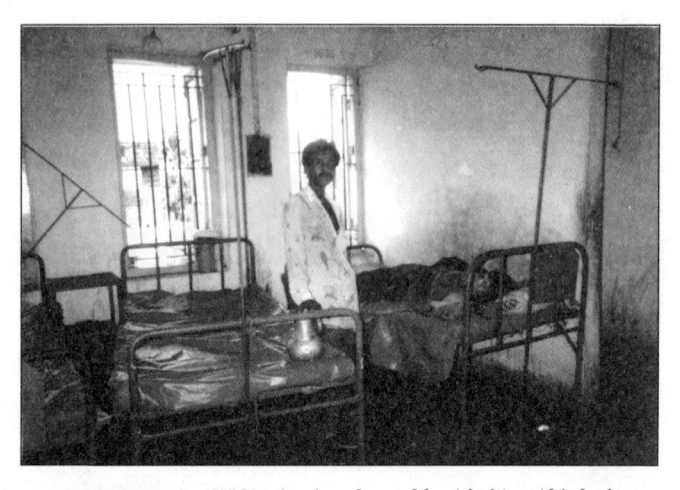

Photo 5: In the THC, a husband stood beside his wife's bed

annoyed at seeing the *ayah* resuscitating the baby. The doctor instructed the second nurse to do resuscitation. The second nurse came forward very reluctantly. She did not seem to know how to resuscitate. Meanwhile, the baby started to cry. The doctor left the room. The *ayah* then went back to the baby and tied the cord. The baby was not weighed. The *ayah* wrapped up the baby with a piece of ragged cloth. One of the relatives took the baby in her lap.

In the meantime, the placenta was expelled out and the bleeding was quite heavy. The nurses asked for more medicines. The second nurse gave another list of medicines to the female relatives. Now, they started a new saline. The first nurse began to joke with the old *daini* who was known to all hospital staff, "How much will you get from this girl Tk. 1500 or 2000?" *Daini* said, "Not a single hollow coin. I wish I could be as rich as you." The nurse asked *daini* to pour water over her hands. *Daini* afterwards told me that nurses always teased her about earning money. The first nurse repaired the episiotomy incision and the tear. Rahena looked exhausted and pale. All the birth substances were left in a bucket. The female sweeper and a female relative changed her petticoat and *saree*. The female sweeper did the entire cleaning job for which she was paid later.

Some male and female relatives along with children waited outside to see the newly born baby. The female relative came out holding the baby in her chest. They all looked happy. Another woman took the baby in her lap. One child was very eagerly observing the baby. The baby seemed hungry. One woman said, "One should get something for Rahena to eat. Get her tea and bread." A male relative went to the market.

Rahena was brought to the female ward. The bed was covered with a plastic sheet. The female sweeper eventually brought a bed linen and a pillow. Rahena lay down on the bed. The baby was put beside her. One male relative brought tea, banana and bread. They all ate together. Rahena and her mother insisted on going back home. Before leaving, they gave some money to the nurses and the *ayah*. *Daini* afterward said, "I told the nurses, please take whatever they can pay, and please buy some sweets. They are poor. I knew that they had paid Tk. 300." Later, in the afternoon, they left the THC.

I went to Rahena's house on the fifth day of her childbirth. She sat on a *chowki*. The baby was sleeping on the bed. They observed the period of confinement, which would continue till the seventh day. On the seventh day, the *choditula* ceremony would be observed to remove the impurity of birth. From the outset, Rahena was very much reluctant to go to the hospital, especially to avoid male doctors and surgery, but she had to face both. She smiled while I was talking with her. Voicing with other women, Rahena said, "It is good to have baby at home."

Birth in the Medical College Hospital: Shahanara's Experience

Nearly four decades after the establishment of the Medical College Hospital I carried out my fieldwork there. When I reflect on my memories of fieldwork, all the events flash on my mind. One evening, I was passing through the corridor of antenatal wards at the hospital. Like any other day or time, I heard the cracking noises of heavy wheels going along the hospital corridors and veranda. A trolley carrying a birthing woman stopped in front of the antenatal check-up room. I also stopped with them. A special *ayah* pushing the trolley handed over the patient to another special *ayah* and told her in whispering voice, "Poor patient! Be careful! Do not let them get trapped in the clutches of hospital *dalal* (tout or cheat)." Shahanara, the birthing woman, was taken inside the check-up room and moved to a patient examination table. Two elderly women holding each other's hand were accompanying her. The room was very stuffy with no windows. A long curtain screened the door to maintain the privacy of women. A few other patients were lying on the other tables. Some female attendants were standing here and there. Special *ayahs* were sitting on the floor and waiting for patients. Their numbers perhaps exceeded the total number of patients and attendants.

One intern female doctor appeared to examine Shahanara, who was lying down on the examination table. She exposed her abdomen by removing the end of her *saree* and then did a vaginal examination. The doctor suddenly looked confused. She immediately called the clinical assistant to confirm the diagnosis. The clinical assistant examined and said, "It is a case of transverse lie with cord prolapse. The cord is still pulsating. She needs immediate caesarean section." She left the room. The intern doctor told Shahanara's attendants, "I am giving *tumi* (you)[14] a list of medicine. Get it immediately. Otherwise we can't save the baby and the mother." The intern doctor was a young girl. I observed her use of the word *tumi* with these women, which seemed very derogatory. Yet, it was not an uncommon practice among doctors in this hospital. Shahanara's mother was shocked after learning the costs of medicine, "I don't have that much money." She requested the doctor to help her out. The doctor became furious and rudely told her, "Have I opened a free medicine shop? Go and get your medicine. Don't stand up here. Why are you waiting? Do you want me to go to the store and buy your medicine?" After handing the medicine list, she left. Shahanara looked very helpless, but was not nervous.

Shahanara's mother shed tears. She requested all the special *ayahs* embracing their legs, "Please buy me medicine with this money. Get me some medicine on credit." She was about to give her money to an *ayah*. An *ayah* said, "Many women asked us to buy medicine, but afterwards they don't pay us back. We are also poor, who will sell us medicine on credit?" Another *ayah* added, "Do you want us to marry a drug seller? We don't care about you. Collect your money by yourself." Everyone was passing more or less similar remarks.

Let me briefly recount why and how Shahanara arrived at the hospital with her mother and mother-in-law. Shahanara, a young girl of 18 and a primigravida, started labour pain the previous evening. A *daini* was called. Shahanara had stronger pain, but the baby's head was not coming down. *Daini* later on announced, "Baby's head is not showing up. Its head is on one side of the abdomen and the feet on the other side. Take her to the hospital." On the following morning, she was taken to the THC, which was two to three kilometres away from their residence. In the THC, the doctors kept her waiting for four to five hours. Shahanara's brother went back home to get food. Meanwhile, one doctor told them to immediately transfer her to the nearest Chikonmati hospital that provides good services to the poor. Shahanara along with her mother and mother-in-law took a *tempo* and went to that hospital. She was not able to get admission into this hospital, as the admission was closed for some reasons. The two elderly women decided to take her to the Medical College Hospital. Shahanara's mother said, "I can't let her die. Going back home means – she will die." They reached the hospital on a public bus with the help of the bus driver.

Shahanara needed medicine immediately. Two elderly women were helpless and cried holding each other. One *ayah* said, "We can't buy your medicine. Get it by yourself." They came out and moved towards the opposite direction. I asked them, "Do you know the drugstore?" "No mother, we don't know anything here," they said. I said, "Let me help you." I told the mother-in-law to stay with Shahanara, but she held Shahanara's mother tightly and started crying, "No, I can't stay here alone." I said, "Alright! We will all go together." They hesitated to go with me. If they moved one step forward, they moved back two steps. I again persuaded them to follow me. I asked them, "How much money do you have?" "I brought Tk. 600 with me," she said. I gave her Tk. 700. She was very surprised, "Mother, people like you also exist in this world. In these days, does anyone give money? Perhaps the God has sent you." I told her, "Don't worry. Keep this money carefully." A special *ayah* was passing by. She stopped and listened to us. I requested her to accompany them to the drugstore. Both of the women got frightened. The *ayah* said, "Come with me. If not, hospital touts will cheat you." She showed them how to keep the money safely. Again, they started to cry. I explained the situation and went back to the antenatal room. After a while, the two women ran and returned to the antenatal check-up room. I said, "What's the matter?" One of them said, "If we can't find our daughter, what will happen then?" They insisted on the special *ayah* buying the medicine for them. Then, I tried to convince one to stay and the other to accompany the *ayah*. Shahanara's mother said, "I am feeling very exhausted. My body is becoming numb. I can't go." The mother-in-law held the mother tightly. The special *ayah* got annoyed and forced the mother-in-law to stay with Shahanara. The mother-in-law entered into the room crying.

Shahanara's mother and the special *ayah* came back with the medicine. The *ayah* did not spend all the money. She said, "You may need some money for buying blood." Both the elderly women blessed my family and me. The doctors took the medicine and prepared Shahanara for caesarean section. Within half an hour, all of them started towards the operating theatre. At that time, both the women went back to the room where Shahanara waited. They picked up their bags. Meanwhile, the special *ayahs* took their daughter to operating theatre. When they came out, the two women screamed, "Where did they take our patient?" They ran through the corridor and looked to the left and right to get hold of their daughter.

Meanwhile, I visited the labour room, which seemed to be less crowded. One intern female doctor was conducting the delivery of a woman whose perineum was fully exposed. Six to seven male and female students were standing there. A unit registrar who happened to be a male doctor was teaching students about different stages of labour. The intern doctor continually dilated the birth passage of the labouring woman with gloved hands. The unit registrar also did a vaginal examination to show the progress of labour to the students. This woman came from a poor family. Her female relative was standing on her right side. The saline drip was attached to her right hand. One special *ayah* was assisting the intern doctor. Her perineum was bulging. The intern doctor gave episiotomy incision on the perineal area. The registrar was describing the process of episiotomy incision. The baby was delivered out and its cry was feeble. It was handed to the *ayah* who started to resuscitate the baby. After removing the placenta, the intern doctor put cotton balls inside the woman's vagina, and later joined the *ayah*. The baby continued crying but still sounded feeble. The woman's perineal area was covered with blood. Another special *ayah* gave a hand to clean the birth substances. The woman's private parts still remained exposed. Suddenly, I noticed that none of the nurses were in the labour room, and later found them in nurses' duty room chatting with each other.

I moved to the operating theatre where Shahanara along with her mother and mother-in-law and the special *ayah* were waiting. The *ayah* came toward me, "We need to buy more medicine. Please check the list." Shahanara was sitting on a bed. After a while, a doctor came out and Shahanara was taken in. The mother-in-law tried to enter into the operating theatre, but was not allowed in. Both of them sat on the floor and started to cry again. They were asked to sit on the bed. Shahanara's mother looked bit happier. She said, "My son arrived. He brought food from home. He didn't know that we came here. He first looked for us at the THC, then at Chikonmati hospital and now, found us here." They all blessed me again and promised to pay back my money as soon as possible.

On the following day, I met Shahanara's mother and mother-in-law in the corridor sitting with the newborn baby. As soon as they saw me, both mentioned returning my money. I felt embarrassed. Did they think I am a creditor? I wanted to see Shahanara in the post-operative ward, but was hesitant to walk over the dirty, muddy, wet floor. It was the weekly cleansing day of the hospital. Both of the women walked happily over the wet floor. The mother was anxious about her son's return, "My son has yet to come back with money. I don't know when they will ask for more medicine." We were sitting outside the post-operative room. The mother became very emotional while sharing her daughter's story,

> I thought, once we reached hospital, some arrangements would be made. But, that's not true. Doctors do not do anything. You need money for treatment. Doctors do not want to listen, but become irritated. The government has made this hospital to suck money from the patients. If patients do not come to the hospital, do you think it will run? Hospitals run on people's money, but they do not get any treatment.

I vigilantly listened to her narrative regarding the current hospital practices. Poor, rural women usually maintained silence about their problems.

I entered into the post-operative room. Most beds were occupied. Shahanara was half-asleep opened her eyes. I told her to have a good sleep. A woman lying on the next bed said, "She was snoring the whole night." This woman happened to be an intern doctor's sister. She was admitted with pregnancy complications, but still had not had surgery. In this ward, only postoperative patients are allowed to stay. Due to her relationship with an intern doctor, she was put in this particular room because it was air conditioned and relatively clean. In this room, I met a female intern doctor who was attending the patients. She discussed the difficulties of the doctors to manage rural, poor patients. Referring to this, she commented, "These patients are very strange! If you shout at them, they will buy medicine. It is a regular event happening here. Why do they behave so strange? These women should not conceive if they can't afford."

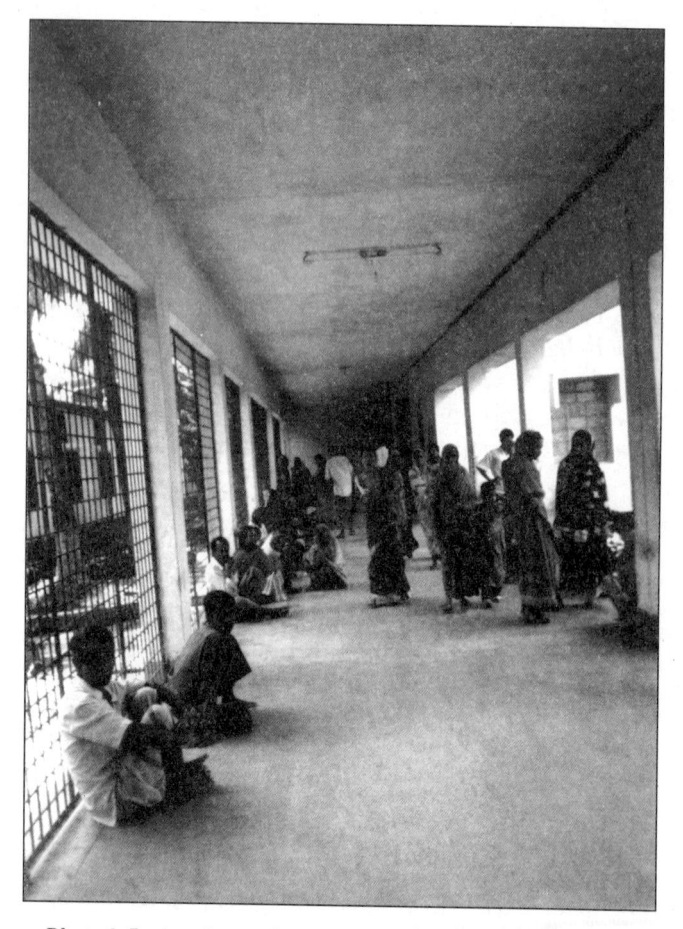

Photo 6: Patients' attendants were waiting in hospital corridor

I continued my discussion with Shahanara's mother. She said,

Nobody values poor people. Everyone is God's servant. Some are rich and some poor. Poor respects rich, but rich does not respect poor. All are made by God and made similar. Then, why is there a difference? If people love each other, God will reward them.

I asked, "Why did you get so panicked yesterday?" She explained,

This is the first time we came here. It is a huge building and we don't know anything. We feared getting lost. Besides, we heard stories of hospital touts. We did not have much money, but we didn't want to lose what we had.

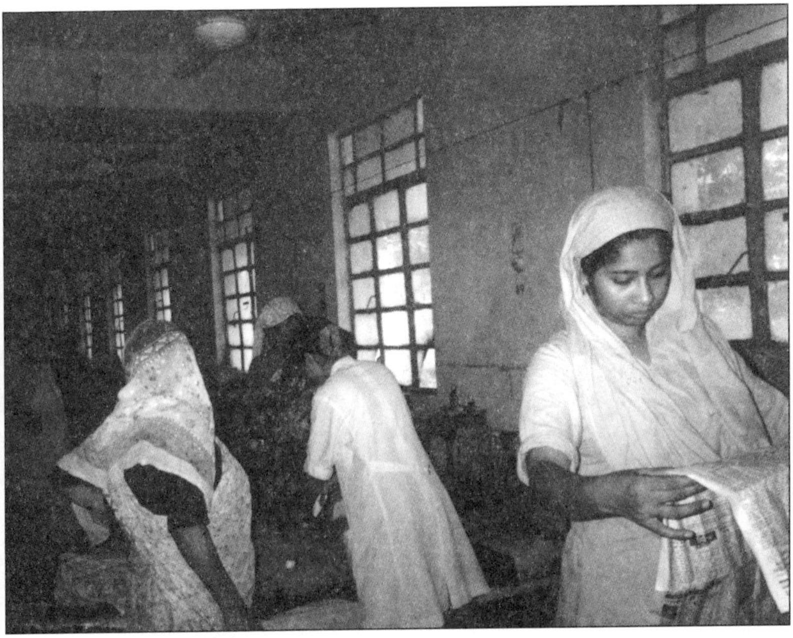

Photo 7: A doctor was examining a patient in a postnatal ward

I met them later in the postnatal ward. Shahanara was lying down on a bed. They seemed very happy to get a bed in the ward. Her mother looked fresh, "I just had a good shower. My daughter's mother-in-law is taking shower now." Shahanara was also given a hair wash. She could not move her left arm because of the saline drip. The baby was placed on her right arm. Her mother was trying to put the nipple in the baby's mouth. She said, "Nurses do not want to come. If you call them, they will not behave well. They sometimes come with one or two medicines. For setting the saline drip, you have to run after them." I found nurses talking in their room. They busied themselves with maintaining medicine registers and counting bed-sheets and blankets.

Two doctors were attending the patients. They were refreshing the daily treatment order. None of them talked to the patients unless they were asked questions. They looked fairly tired. Shahanara said, "These two doctors are nice." I entered into the doctor's room attached to the ward. It was more than 1 pm. The intern doctor asked me to sit with her.

She was writing discharge certificates. The doctor said, "Our madam[15] (head of the unit) will be very unhappy if she finds out that we are writing discharge certificates so late." After writing the certificates, she explained to the patients or their attendants. Yet, this was not a common picture of patient's discharge. Most patients and their attendants had bitter experiences in getting discharge certificates.

Shahanara left the hospital on the ninth day after her operation. She did not have trouble on discharge from the hospital. I went to visit her after a month at her village home. Shahanara lived about 30 kilometres away from the Medical College Hospital. On our discussion about hospital experiences, she commented,

> I feared at the beginning because I never had such experiences before. I never went to hospital before. I was scared because I came to the hospital for the first time. When I was referred from the THC, I was very frightened. I didn't have enough money. No men accompanied us. I don't know anyone. I don't know what will be done to me. I had to be brave enough to take decisions. Here, doctors don't communicate if you can't buy medicine. I would have died if you were not there. You are dead if you have no money to buy medicine. We spent about Tk. 8000 for my treatment. We had to take loan from a moneylender who charged very high interest rate. It is difficult to arrange so much money within such a short time. Otherwise, doctors and nurses did not behave badly. They let me sleep on the bed. They gave me two bags of saline free. What else do you expect?

Her interpretations of hospital experiences seemed self-critical and self-denying. I observed her experiences and the medical treatment she obtained in the hospital. Even then, she expressed her gratitude to doctors for getting her life back blessed with a little daughter, "I am thankful to them. After all, they saved my life." Her mother echoed her voice with her daughter saying, "We must thank them."

3.3 SUMMARY AND CONCLUSION

In presentations of two contemporary birth practices, my observational experiences combine with women's voices. In indigenous birthing practices, the description was of a typical portrayal of birth experience in a village. The birth event was accomplished by the participation of the birthing women along with the *daini* and others. Raheemon was quite confident in giving birth. With own understandings of bodily experiences and mutual communications with the *daini* and other women, she gave birth without much discomfort. *Daini* did play a significant role by using her indigenous knowledge and skills. Women kept the environment of birth event lively by sharing their knowledge.

This also boosted up Raheemon. The birth event was surrounded by social norms and practices, which were actually part of their everyday life.

In the hospital, experiences of Rahena and Shahanara were not atypical. In fact, some were more complex. These women had to go through a range of experiences in facing doctors, nurses and the other hospital staff. Biomedical professionals exercised power over women's birth experiences. It was observed in Rahena's birth event, which was controlled by the nurses in the THC. She had very little to do while giving birth. In the Medical College Hospital, Shahanara was not aware of her birth experience, as she had undergone caesarean section. The costs of hospital treatment and experiences of unfamiliar environment were quite traumatic. The interplay of different individuals created a situation, which was not congenial to women's birth experiences in hospitals.

In sum, women's birth experience in hospitals was very different from that of home. Yet, in either of the systems, we can see that the understandings and participations of different individuals influence the construction of birth. The following chapters will deconstruct aspects of indigenous and cosmopolitan birth practices in order to arrive at a series of recommendations that draw on the strengths of each system of knowledge and practice.

Notes

[1] The concept of cosmopolitan medicine was first introduced by Frederick L. Dunn in Charles Leslie's *Asian Medical Systems: A Comparative Study* in order not to limit its meaning to modern, western, scientific medicine (Dunn, 1976; Leslie, 1976). Introduced for the benefits of comparison among different practices of health care locally or regionally, cosmopolitan medicine actually referred to modern biomedicine that originated in the western world but took on different shapes and meanings in other countries as a consequence of socio-cultural, political and global influences (Leslie, 1976). In modern/traditional dichotomy, modernity assumes a changing and creative nature, whereas traditionalism represents a stagnant and unchanging position. However, considerable changes have occurred in the last century in so-called 'traditional' medicine. Chinese and Indian medicines have attracted worldwide attention due to their innovations

and research, and incorporations into a modern system of health care. These traditions are also substantially scientific as they involve rational use of naturalistic theories to organise and interpret systematic empirical observations. On the other hand, all aspects of cosmopolitan medicine are not scientific, for example, the politics of research funding, or of professional associations, various routines of hospital administrations or of the etiquette of doctor-patient relationship. It is no more a Western medicine because its scientific aspects and social organisation are transcultural (Dunn, 1976; Leslie, 1976).

2 *Daiburi* means an old *dai* used in my home town, which is located in the Northern part of Bangladesh.

3 It is an Arabic month when Muslims perform fasting from the sunrise to sunset.

4 *Korkora bhat* is leftover cold, stiff rice from last night's meal.

5 The local word, *sharam* is directly translated to Bangla word, *sharam*. In most literatures, the Bangla word, '*sharam*' is directly translated to shame, which has very much negative connotations in English. It is a word not to indicate negative feelings of rural women in their attitudes to pregnancy and childbirth related issues. In fact, rural women view *sharam* as being shy or bashful and something relating to modesty. The usage of *sharam* may vary with the context and hence, its meaning sometimes may change from shyness to shame. At this point, I am much concerned with its usage and how it works in the socio-cultural context. The word, '*sharam*' is used all through to directly transmit women's message to readers.

6 *Chodi* means pollution and *ghar* room. *Chodighar* is the seclusion room set for birthing mother, as she is considered polluted.

7 *Kajol* is black soot prepared by heating *khodar gourur haar* or any metal objects over the flames of clay made lamp lighted with mustard oil.

8 *Khodar gorur haar* is literally translated to God's cow bone. It is in fact a piece of cow bone where the cow is specifically sacrificed on a religious festival of Muslims known as Eid-Ul-Azha.

9 *Choditula* is a local word, which means removal of pollution.

10 A bamboo made horseshoe shaped plate is used for winnowing rice.

11 *Matir prodip* is a clay-made flat lamp used in worshipping God and Goddess among Hindus.

12 *Khur* is an iron made knife used for shaving hair. It is considered sacred because the water dipped with *khur* is sprinkled inside and around the birthing house for purification.

13 *Chowki* is a wooden flat, elevated bed with four legs.

14 In Bengali language, the word 'you' is translated to *apni*, *tumi* and *tui*. *Apni* is used specifically with seniors to show respects, *tumi* with same aged persons, like spouses and friends and siblings, and *tui* with friends and juniors, like children, siblings and relatives. The use of word 'you' also is dependent on the relationship. Bangladeshi society is very much stratified by social status. Thus, the word 'you' is used with caution. Using *tumi* with elderly poor women seemed very derogatory to me.

15 In Bangladesh, all the female teachers are called as 'Madam' as opposed to male teachers who are called as 'Sir'.

Chapter 4

Indigenous Birth Practices: Construction of Birth in *Apurbabari*

As in many developing countries, indigenous practices of childbirth have persisted for generations among people in Bangladesh, particularly in rural areas (Afsana & Rashid, 2000; Blanchet, 1984; Rozario, 1998). Different social norms and practices are observed in indigenous birth (Blanchet, 1984; Rozario, 1998). As a person with previous medical background, I have encountered dilemma to accept the safe performance of indigenous birth practices. However, my field experiences and analytical thinking have shaped my own understandings of the birthing practices. In this chapter, my intention is to present experiences of women, including birthing women, *dainis* and other women who play a crucial role in indigenous birth. My observational experiences strengthen voices heard during fieldwork. I will also describe the role of men and the local healers and heath practitioners, who are directly or indirectly involved in birth event. In the course of description, understanding of childbirths and the social practices will be highlighted. In brief, this chapter moves out from the presentation of one particular birth event to describe the dimensions of indigenous birth practices from multiple perspectives.

4.1 WOMEN IN BIRTHING

A woman is the central figure in indigenous childbirth. Each woman plays a pivotal role by actively participating in her own birth experience. Other women render supports in the birthing process. In this section, the experiences of birthing women and other women in birth events will be discussed.

Understanding of Birth

The rural women understood the birthing process as *thikmoton oiche* (happened exactly how it should be) or *kolbekol oiche* (happened with problems or difficulties). The descriptions of women's understanding suggested that birth should take place without any complications and similar to usual births in this village. As Rownak explicated this issue, "When a woman gives birth like other women in the village, we accept it as a usual birth. As she does not have any problem, childbirth is considered to take place at home." Since birth was expected to happen like other usual births in the village, they all preferred to have birth at home.

Kol-bekol was not an unexpected phenomenon in birth events. It was seen as something dissimilar to the usual birth patterns. When *kolbekol* happened during birthing, or was identified earlier, women still tried to give birth at home. They sought other options, especially hospital care only if the birth trial failed at home. Women believed that *kolbekol* was the God's punishment against committing sin causing sufferings from prolonged labour or breech presentation. Mameena's first childbirth was an *ukta* (breech) presentation that took place at home with the assistance of several *dainis*. She encountered difficulties in giving birth and subsequently developed uterine prolapse. Mameena believed that her breech delivery happened due to the God's punishment, but her postpartum uterine prolapse occurred due to mismanaged birth. Therefore, during her second childbirth, she desperately sought cosmopolitan obstetric care when labour seemed prolonged. One young woman had premature, twin delivery and both her babies died within an hour. The attack of evil wind was blamed for causing her *kolbekol*. As her sister-in-law explained, "She went to her mother's house. On her return in the evening, she was attacked by *batash* (evil wind). After that, she developed slight pain and gave birth much earlier than her due time." Women also related intrauterine death and miscarriage with the attacks of evil spirits and evil spells. To avoid the mishaps, they wore amulets around their neck or arms. Rural women adopted different strategies to cope with the crisis of pregnancy-related problems.

Enduring *Moner Shahosh* and *Shoriler Shakti*

A saying circulated in *Apurbabari* village, "*Baacha houner shomey moner shahosh aar shoriler shakti lagey* (to participate in childbirth experiences, one needs to have mental strength and physical vigour)." The rural women put emphasis on the two issues in order to have a normal birth, one was *moner shahosh* and the other was *shoriler shakti*. In reference to that, Marsheeda said, "If birthing women are not mentally and physically strong, they won't be able to give birth by themselves." The relationship of *moner shahosh* and *shoriler shakti* with psychological and physiological experiences was reflected in the words of Tohmeena, "Your mental strength arises from your mind and your physical strength from your body." Women believed that this knowledge influenced them to understand their bodily mechanisms and enabled them to give birth. For example, Raheemon observed, "Only if you have *moner shahosh* and *shoriler shakti*, you can correlate your labour pain with the downward movement of the baby and understand when to push." On the other hand, Kamila, a *daini*, added, "If women do not sustain *moner shahosh* and *shoriler shakti*, they lose their *disha* (sense) during the birth event and become confused with labour pain and the movement of foetus."

This knowledge was circulating among the rural women for generations. The rural women acquired the knowledge of *moner shahosh* and *shoriler shakti* from other women, such as their mother, grandmother, sisters, relatives, neighbours, and *dainis*. Each of these women encouraged birthing women to sustain their knowledge. A young girl of sixteen, who I met in the antenatal care centre said, "My sister-in-law told me to keep *moner shahosh* and *shorlier shakti*, otherwise I won't be able to give birth at home." It was observed that previous birth experiences also had an effect on developing knowledge. Women knew the importance of having this knowledge, thus, not only they retained it for their own birth experience but also encouraged other birthing women to sustain it. I observed during the birth event of Shagoreen, how Kamila, Feloni and her mother inspired her to actively participate in birthing, "*Money shahosh rakh, shoriley shakti kor* (Endure mental strength and beget physical vigour)." This brought immense strength and confidence to ensure a normal childbirth. Shagoreen said, "I felt much stronger with their words." Nonetheless, the strength women sustained in their own birthing experiences might not remain when they attended other birth events. As one woman said, "I can participate in my own birth, but am not brave enough to see the birth of another child." The context in which women lived influenced them to endure *moner shahosh* and *shoriler shakti* in their own birthing process, however, it might adopt different shapes with the changing context.

Moner shahosh and *shoriler shakti* were seen to influence each other. The women considered the psychological and bodily experiences of childbirth as a collective power. They felt that if mental strength was deficient, the physical vigour could not act alone. Referring to her sister, Hafizan said, "She has *nirjhori* (emaciated) body. How will she deliver the baby? Despite her *moner shahosh*, she does not have *shoriler shakti* to push down." On the other hand, Papreen, lacking mental strength, was not able to give birth at home in spite of her physical vigour. Women understood that the two forces worked together and acted on birthing women to bring about a normal birth. Thus, the collective power of psychosomatic experiences was considered crucial to procreate a new life.

The indigenous knowledge of *moner shahosh* and *shoriler shakti* can be affected by external reasons obscuring women's active role in giving birth. Women experiencing their first birth or having previous birth mishaps were seen to possess very little *moner shahosh* to participate in birth events. Educated women in the village seeking hospital obstetric care were also blamed for not having enough *moner shahosh*. Similarly, some women in the village believed that the birthing women who willingly participated in local, safe motherhood programmes lost their *moner shahosh* to give birth at home. For example, Hamida and Humayra, two community health workers of the local NGO, and Mameena, an active member of the NGO community-based health programme, went to the local THC as soon as they developed prolonged labour. They were seen to possess little *moner shahosh* due to their involvement with the NGO-run health programme. Conversely, *shoriler shakti* was lessened among malnourished women, particularly those who experienced multiple births.

The women also understood that with increasing age and number of births, *moner shahosh* was reinforced and their active participation in birth events was enhanced, but, *shoriler shakti* was diminished. With the reduced *shoriler shakti*, experienced women were occasionally unable to give birth at home and sought hospital care. As Feloni, a *daini*, stated, "*Boyosh barle addi batti oi. Baccha ouner shomey khulse na* (Bones become hardened as one gets older. It won't open up during child delivery)." With increasing age, pelvic joints were thought to lose elasticity that also made older women to participate in birth events less successfully.

INDIGENOUS BIRTH PRACTICES 67

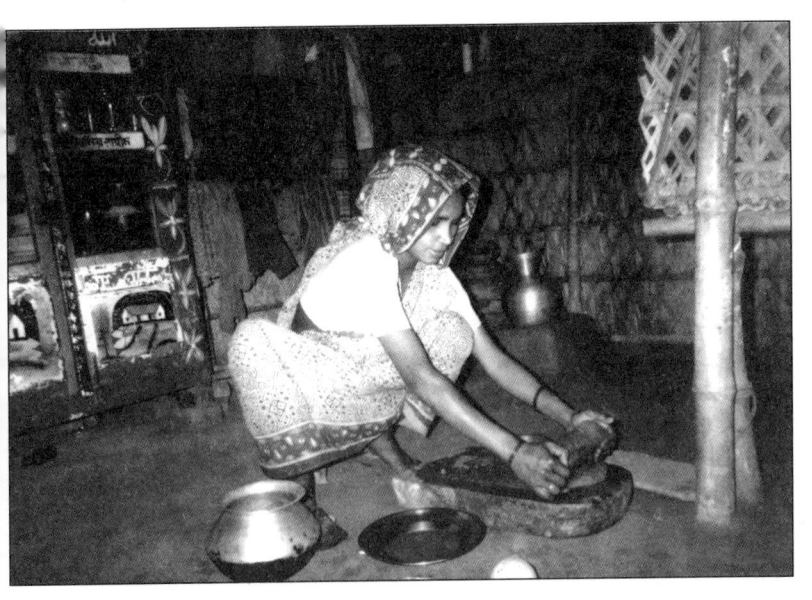

Photo 8: Hashima was grinding spices the day before her labour pain

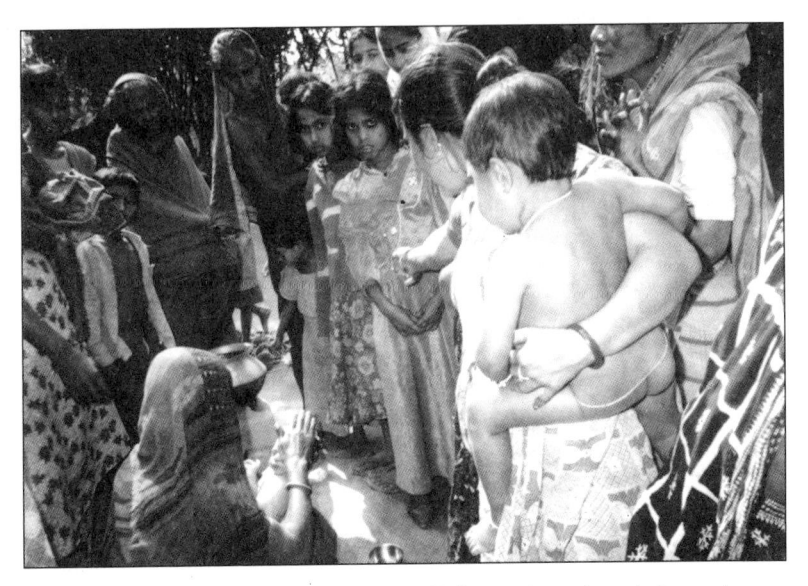

Photo 9: Ambika was giving bath to Raheemon's newborn baby, and Taljan, the daini was watching the event along with the neighbours

Halema, 32 years old, became pregnant after 16 years of marriage. The local *daini* said, "She conceived at *pura kale* (matured age) and had prolonged labour for two days. Then, we took her to the hospital. They delivered the baby after cutting her birth passage." Older women were, therefore, considered to develop problems during pregnancy.

During the birth events, young women and women with little *moner shahosh* were constantly given emotional support to reinforce it. The woman attending the birth events primarily shared their birth stories to strengthen mental strength of birthing women. I observed a *daini* singing during the birth event. Later she said, "Didn't you see her face? It became shrivelled in fear. I wanted to cheer her up." The birthing women were also asked to call the name of almighty Allah and given *panipora* (sanctified water) to reinstate their *moner shahosh*. In some extreme cases, *dainis* started to recite surahs from the Koran to restore her own mental strength along with that of birthing women and the others. Besides, birthing women were given food to be energised, and to successfully participate in their birth event. They were given warm rice mixed with mustard oil and green chillies. I saw Tohmeena and Raheemon fed freshly cooked warm rice, even though they were not in a mood of eating. The understanding was that eating food reinstated physical energy and compelled birthing women to eat more, in spite of their lack of appetite.

Even with their knowledge of giving birth, women sometimes could not absolutely count on it. Hashima and her mother-in-law became very much worried about her imminent birth event, because she developed urinary retention a few days before her expected date of delivery. Hashima argued, "You may have *moner shahosh* and *shoriler shakti*, but, you may not be able to give normal birth at home because you are facing *kol-bekol* (problems in pregnancy)." Despite *moner shahosh* and *shorliler shakti* women believed that in *kol-bekol* childbirth, experiencing birth at home with assistance from *dainis* might further aggravate the situation. Hence, inability to participate in complicated childbirth and inadequate skills of *dainis* to manage complications gave rise to uncertainty about birth consequences forcing women to consider hospital obstetric care.

Understanding Bodily Mechanisms in Pregnancy and Childbirth

Women had their own understandings of bodily changes during pregnancy and bodily mechanisms in childbirth. Cessation of menstruation, nausea and vomiting, changes in food habits, breast changes, and alterations in sleep patterns were embodied knowledge felt by pregnant women. This knowledge was developed through sharing and listening to other women and through their own understandings of body. By sharing with an aunt, Hamida came to know about her own conception,

> I was not sure of my conception. I felt something different in my body. My menstruation has always been irregular. I was able to eat everything. What is wrong with my body then? I talked to Aunt Sharnarupa, a local *daini*. She is an experienced woman and advised me to squeeze my nipple to look for yellowish fluid. I followed her instructions and found yellowish fluid at the top of my nipple. I felt very happy to know that I was pregnant.

Raheemon added different experience, "When I conceived the first time, I had a different feeling. I was not able to eat anything. This time I felt something different in my body. I was not able to sleep and was always tired." Marsheeda felt some bodily changes during her first conception at very young age,

> I was young and just started my *mashik* (menstrual period) a few months ago. I could not understand my first conception. I was having few drops of bleeding as my *mashik*. But, I felt changes in my breast. My mother-in-law found changes in me and enquired about my physical condition. She said, you are pregnant, my daughter.

This indigenous knowledge acquired from experiences and circumstances was of great value for pregnancy identification.

The understanding of bodily mechanisms enabled women to participate in their own birth experiences. While giving birth, the women felt and understood the movement of the foetus and the progress of labour. Some also understood their progress of labour to such an extent that they prepared themselves accordingly. Tohmeena shared her previous birth experiences,

> When I was ready, I told my sister-in-law about my labour pain. Whenever I felt severe pain, I went inside my bedroom. I knew when to push. I pushed a few times and the baby was born without any hassles.

The women with previous birth experiences were more skilled in understanding the bodily mechanisms during labour, but the women having first birth experience had greater difficulty to understand it.[1] The knowledge of bodily changes arose from their experiential knowledge. Raheemon, a woman giving her second birth told me, "My legs were shivering. I understood my time had come. I felt my baby was coming down *chiryae chuitya* (rushing and tearing down)." During the birth event, she also directed her grandmother Taljan, a *daini* to press her anus, "Please put pressure over my *putki* (anus)." Raheemon was feeling the head of the foetus pressing over her anus. On occasion, birthing women tried to feel the head of the foetus by touching the birth canal and bore down with the intensity of labour pain. The understanding of bodily processes begot both physical and psychological strength that enabled birthing women to actively participate. Being physically weak, Tohmeena commented on her recent birth experience,

> I was able to understand my baby coming down, but my body was too weak to bear down. My mother and sister-in-law became worried. They told me to get *moner shahosh* and *shorlier shakti* and showed me to take squatting posture. I thought, I had to bring the baby out. I squatted. With all *moner shahosh* and s*horiler shakti,* I pushed down firmly and the baby came out.

The active role in birth events was, thus, associated with the psychological and physiological experiences of birthing women.

With the understanding of bodily mechanisms, the birthing women chose to continue free movement, and to adopt birthing postures. Even when they sensed labour pain, they did not refrain from doing normal chores. Although, some women shared doing heavy chores, I observed birthing women performing regular household chores at a slow pace. Marium, a silversmith, who gave birth at night, was seen doing silverworks in the evening. Tohmeena shared her experience,

> I sensed mild pain in the morning. I felt that I should finish preparing meals before starting strong pain. I put rice on the *chula* in the courtyard. My sister-in-law noticed me. She said, go to your room. I will look after your food. I went back to my bed. Then, I came back and cut some vegetables. My pain was becoming stronger. I called my mother-in-law and told her, *ma* please call someone. I am having labour pain. I understood my pain was growing stronger. I entered into the kitchen that we had decided earlier would be my birthing room.

Even during the birth event, birthing women did not restrict their movements. I observed them walking in between their pains, sitting on flat wooden stool and resting on the bed. They were not restricted from going to the toilet when required.

Birthing women adopted different postures by choice. When they felt severe pain, a preferred birthing posture was adopted. I observed in birth events that three women took on a sitting down posture. Two of them leaned over other women and the other one embraced bamboo poles behind. Another adopted a squatting position and grabbed a bamboo pole at the front. However, if labour seemed prolonged, women attending the event conversed with each other and suggested suitable postures to hasten the labour process. During her birth experience, Praveena was asked to kneel down despite the fact that she was not comfortable with it. As her labour became prolonged, the *daini* asked her to change position from semi-recumbent to kneeling down to hasten the process.

Commemorating After-Birth

While the rest of the family celebrated the birth of a newly born, the birthing women sat alone after giving birth. The women who were the centres of attraction during the birth event lost it as soon as the baby was born and the placenta expelled. The women attending the event became busy with the newly born baby. The event that took place so secretly suddenly became public. Women relatives and neighbours and children anxiously waited outside to see the baby. When Sumaiya, the newly born baby was brought out of the room, the women and children became delighted at her sight. Feloni, the *daini*, took the baby first to her paternal grandmother, who was praying on her bed. As the baby had not yet had a bath, she was blessed from afar. In most cases, warm water was used to bathe babies, but, Feloni did not use water. She massaged the baby with mustard oil to remove the birth substances. In this regard, she said, "This will keep her warm. I saw this in the hospital. They clean baby's body by massaging oil." Feloni wrapped up the baby nicely with old clothes and took her around the neighbourhood to show the elders for their blessings. Sumaiya's grandmother said, "The blessings she has received from the elders will make her long-lived and strong." Finally, the baby was brought back to her mother.

Women relatives and neighbours passed different remarks about baby's features and compared her resemblance with other family members. They also blamed the baby for giving suffering to her mother, "You have given lots of troubles to your mother for coming to this world." Sumaiya's grandmother was unhappy to see a baby girl. Afterward she told me, "Look at my three daughters. They couldn't live with their husbands. I don't like other girls to go through the miseries that my daughters faced. I don't feel happy when a baby girl is born." On the other hand, Sumaiya's mother put a different view,

> I am very happy that she is a girl. Now, we don't have to think of dividing the house when they grow up. My two sons will be able to live in this house. We will marry off our daughters and buy them some land in other places.

Shagoreen was very happy with her newly born daughter. As she stated,

> I am very pleased to have a baby girl. I am fed up with my two sons. They are always on the roof or at the top of the tree. My other girl is very nice. Hopefully, this one will be as nice as her.

The other three women whose birth event I observed were happy with the biological sex of their babies. They commented: Allah has given us the baby that we expected.

Leaving birthing women unaccompanied right after birth made me curious. I asked Raheemon and Hashima about their feelings whey they were left alone after giving birth. Both of them simply looked at me. They were confused, as they could not understand my question. Hashima said, "Oh! I needed to take a bath to clean myself." Another woman commented on it, "That's how it happens in this village." I explained to women about the afterbirth consequences of mothers much later when I finished my fieldwork. They said, "We never thought about it before. You are right. We know that many women die after giving birth."

All the birthing women usually took a bath to cleanse them after the baby was born. If it happened during daytime, they took bath immediately. Warm water was used for bathing purpose. I touched bath water in Raheemon's birth event to feel its temperature. It was a very cold day in winter and water was reasonably cold. Elderly women sometimes insisted on giving bath to mother and baby even when the birth took place at night. Ambika, 50 years old commented on this, "My first child was born in a very cold winter night. They gave bath to the baby with cold water. Next day, he became blue and died. I don't like when people want to give a bath at night." After taking a bath, women changed clothes wearing very old petticoats and a blouse and covered the upper body with a ragged *saree* or old shawl. The baby was placed on mother's lap for breastfeeding. The birthing women waited outside until a place was set for the period of confinement.

Although, the baby was kept till the seventh day inside the hut to protect them from supernatural forces, visitors were not restricted to enter into the room and to hold the baby. Hashima said, "We can't displease them. After all, they are *mehman* (guest). It is important to have their blessings on the baby." After the *choditula* ceremony, especially after shaving hair and removing finger and toenails, the baby became part of the community to adapt and survive. A typical comment was: The baby needs to be *shokto-mokto* (strong and sturdy). During my stay in the village, I saw all the babies whose births I had witnessed roaming around the village in the lap and on the shoulders of other children, women and men.

Celebrating birth by distributing sweets[2] was an unusual event in this village. Most people were poor and spending money on sweets was a luxury. After Raheemon's son was born, children demanded sweets from the family, but it did not eventuate. I noticed Tohmeena's husband buying sweets for the family and neighbours on the day of *choditula*. Tohmeena did not like this, "*Apa*, look at my husband. He does not have any job. What is the point of spending so much money in distributing sweets? He said that people would bless our son." We were also offered sweets. I felt guilty for eating this sweet, as Tohmeena's family did not have much money to buy their regular meals.

Feeling *Sharam*

Sharam was a social norm commonly practiced in the everyday life of rural women. Disclosing the news of being pregnant was a matter of *sharam*, specifically for the women who had conceived for the first time. Women primarily came to know the feelings associated with conception from their socialisation and circumstantial experiences. When women first conceived, they never disclosed the news to others. Woman family members observing changes in a newly pregnant woman's behaviour discussed the matter among them. Women whispered among themselves until pregnancy became visible. As the issues of pregnancy were kept secret, sometimes their problems remained unnoticed. I met Karimon who was accidentally discovered as pregnant. As her conception was suddenly revealed, Rownak, a neighbouring woman laughed at and teased her. This young girl of 17 was three months pregnant. She spoke with me about her occasional, slight bleeding. I advised her to communicate with the community health workers and the THC. Rownak said, "This bleeding is normal.

Any woman could have this. It will go away." Unfortunately, it did not cease. Karimon had a miscarriage after a few days, which was also kept hidden.

Sharam was felt when pregnancy became visible. Women tried to hide pregnancy from men by covering their abdomen with one end of their *saree*. One Hamida said, "People will call you shameless if you walk around keeping your abdomen uncovered." Some women even refrained from visiting natal home to avoid the sight of their own father and brother during pregnancy period. Hamida said, "I can't go to my father's house. How will I face my father, brother and uncles with my bulky abdomen? They will also feel shy." But, on the contrary rural women used to breastfeed by exposing their breasts even in the presence of strange men without feeling *sharam*. I observed women taking a bath with neighbouring men in the same pond by exposing their upper body. When I raised questions about these issues, the women seemed confused and laughed at me.

In rural societies, birthing is a secret matter. A proverb sustained in this village was, "*Joto rao hobe, toto deri hobe baccha houne aar toto koshto hobe* (the more people talk about the birth event, the more time it requires and the more suffering occurs when giving birth)." Thus, to avoid birthing problems, birth events were observed very secretly in *Apurbabari* village. When labour began, birthing women carried on their daily chores maintaining a painless gesture. The other women in the household also remained silent. They did not even aspire to share this with their male counterparts. Women who were likely to attend the birth event inquired the birthing women about labour progress and simultaneously carried out their daily tasks as if nothing happened. The event was performed so quietly that close female neighbours were sometimes not aware of it. However, Kamila gave an opposing view about the understanding of birth secrecy, "Birth event is performed secretly not to avoid prolonged labour but to avoid a gathering of people." Women bore diverse views on the same issues around the village.

To maintain secrecy during the birth event was very important. During my fieldwork, I became friendly with a family to observe the birth event of their daughter. Their house was very close to my residence. I went to their house one evening. Kalpamoti, a young pregnant woman looked a bit different. I wanted to know her physical state. She said, "Perfectly alright!" Very early in the morning, I heard that someone was knocking at my door. I opened the door and it was

Kalpamoti's grandmother. She was smilingly saying, "Kalpamoti has been blessed with a son last night." I was shocked, but maintained smile, "Why didn't you call me?" She explained that they tried to call me, but did not want the whole *para* to know that Kalpamoti was having labour pain. The house was locked at the front side for security reasons. She would have made it through the back door, but in order to avoid crossing the neighbours' houses, she went back home silently. She said, "*Joto rao hobe, toto deri hobe baccha houne aar toto koshto hobe* (the more people talk about the birth event, the more time it requires and the more suffering occurs when giving birth)." Being a medically trained doctor, I discovered my position worthless and unwanted in the midst of the people's understandings of birth being a private, secret matter. But, being a novice ethnographer, I found their understandings of birth and issues of *sharam* have meanings and implications in their social context.

Enduring pain in silence was commonly observed during childbirth. Birthing women were invariably eulogised for their silence in labour. This cultural expression of pain brought them self-pride.[3] The women wanted their labour process to be quiet and did not intend to express pain unless it became unbearable. Tohmeena said,

> As a woman, you are not supposed to make any noise so that others can hear your cry. A woman should bear pain in silence. I never needed any assistance during my delivery. After awhile my family members heard the cry of the newly born baby. My mother-in-law came in to help me out.

Listening to birthing women's screaming, particularly by men was a matter of extreme *sharam*. By maintaining silence women endured their pain and controlled bodily experiences. As Rownak explained her situation, "I was having a severe headache during my labour pain, but did not tell anyone. Later on, I lost consciousness and was taken to the hospital. At the end, I gave birth to a dead baby." Hence, women's non-expression of problems led to life threatening situations and at times, death of mother and baby.

Sharam was very much related to revealing of private parts. Not only birthing women felt *sharam* to expose their private parts, but *dainis* also tried not to see women's exposed vaginal area. I observed that birthing women covered their perineal area by pulling their petticoat over the legs. Shagoreen in her birth event left her upper body uncovered, but wore a petticoat so as not to expose her perineal area. She was concerned about her nine-year old boy coming to the room. It was very late night and birth took place in their only room. Her son roamed around outside sobbing, "Mom let me come in. I want to sleep." Kamila, a *daini* said, "Let him sleep in." Shagoreen said, "No. He will observe everything." She cautioned other women not to allow him into the room and asked not to bring the lamps close to her perineal area.

Showing *gorvochul* (baby's hair at birth) was considered a matter of *sharam*. The baby's hair was generally shaved on the seventh day to remove birth pollution. But, during my fieldwork, I found one newly born girl's head was shaved on the third day by the *daini* who also attended the birth. I learnt that shaving was done to remove the matter of *sharam*,

> Seeing *gorvochul* is a matter of *sharam*, especially if men see. This hair grows inside the mother's womb, seeing *gorvochul* and women's private part is the same. The baby's father asked me to shave his daughter's hair so that men cannot envisage his wife's private part. It is like committing a sin. More men seeing *gorvochul* means more sin will be committed.

Interestingly, this baby's father was completely unaware of the matter while I discussed this with him. Some of the issues created by women circulated among them, but men had little access to it.

Observing *Chochi* (Pollution)

The observance of pollution rituals varied among families in *Apurbabari* village. Menstrual blood accumulating in the mother's womb for the long '10-month' period was regarded as the source of *chochi*. Women with postpartum bleeding were usually considered dangerously polluted[4], particularly for the first six days of childbirth. As polluted blood was seen to be linked with evil spirits, *chochi* women were liable to cause dangers.[5] People wearing amulets or suffering from diseases were afraid of *chochi*. They understood that the amulet would lose power and their condition would deteriorate if they came in contact with a *chochi* mother. People feared that touch of *chochi* women would cease cows' ability to give milk and destroy paddy field. Thus, *chochi* was avoided till the seventh day of childbirth.

Birthing women were not allowed to touch the *chula* during the period of *chochi*. Women who came into contact with *chochi* women always took a bath before initiating any chores. The woman assisting birthing women sometimes remained secluded. On the seventh day, *choditula*, the ceremony of pollution removal was celebrated where all the rituals of

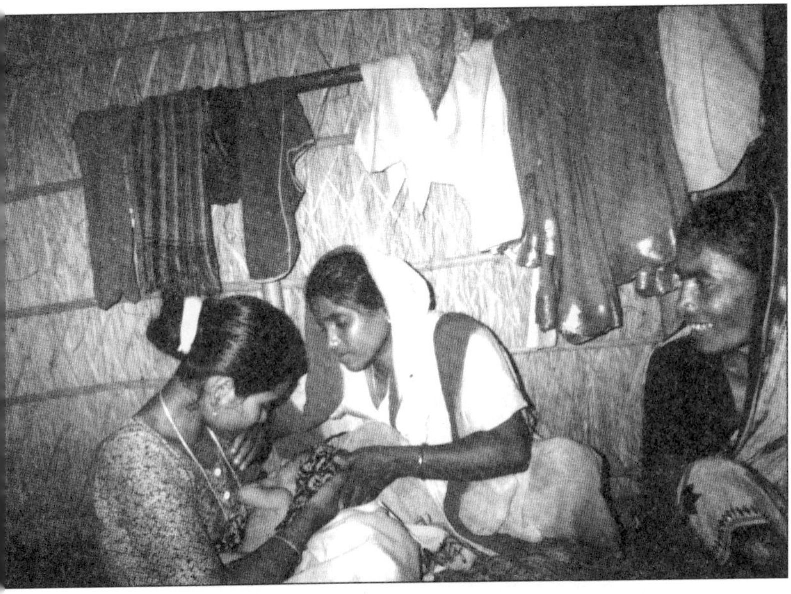

*Photo 10: A mother-in-law was helping the first-time
mother breastfeed the baby. A daini sat beside them*

purification were observed. The birthing women became fully free of *chochi* after 40 days when they were able to perform prayers and observe religious practices. Surprisingly, a baby was not considered as *chochi* as a mother. *Gorvochul* grown in mother's womb was understood to be nourished with menstrual blood, and considered as *chochi*. The baby became completely free of *chochi*, as soon as baby's hair was shaved.

Nevertheless, not everyone strictly observed the norms of *chochi*. Shagoreen was highly criticised by her relatives and neighbours for entering into her uncle's hut on the second day and touching *chula* on the third day. She said, "I was tired of sitting inside my hut and went to my uncle's hut to watch TV." Regarding cooking meals, she strongly stated, "Who will cook for my family?" My discussion with other women revealed that their mothers and grandmothers were not able to observe *chochi* very strictly. In reference to that, one woman stated,

> They were wives of *kolus* (oil-makers). They did not have time to sit around and observe *chochi*. A day or two after childbirth they had to begin their daily chores. They had to help in oil making, which was their business.

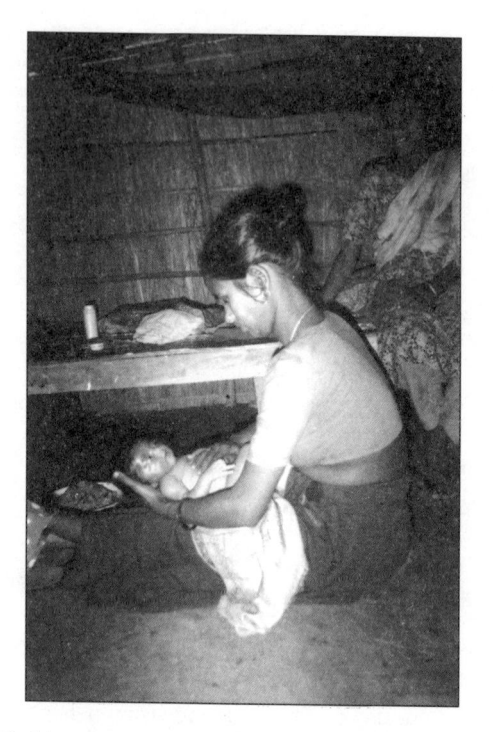

Photo 11: Hashima was massaging the newborn baby with oil in chodighar

The way people observed and reflected on *chochi* varied from family to family. This cultural knowledge had considerable impact on rural women's practices of birthing.

Hydor (Evil Spirit) and *Baobatash* (Evil Wind)

Chochi women were seen to be vulnerable to attacks of *hydor* and *baobatash*. Many rituals were observed till the ceremony of *choditula* to avoid it. In *Apurbabari* village, to prevent the attacks of *hydor*, a bunch of bamboo broomsticks, a few twigs of *nishinda* leaves, a cow-bone, an iron sickle and a small torn part of fishing-net were fastened together to make a bundle. This bundle was kept beside the baby's bed along with a matchbox. Some people also left leather materials, for example, sandal. The newly born baby was carried always with this bundle to keep the *hydor* away. I also observed that Raheemon constantly kept firewood burning for the first six days to avoid the *hydor*.

The birthing women tried to confine themselves within the room till the sixth day. Women were not allowed to go out at mid-day, evening and night when evil spirits were believed to be active. They usually went out only for a bath and for emptying bowel and bladder during daytime. But, they always carried a matchbox. When entering into the room, the birthing women touched their bodies with broomsticks and *nishinda* leaves, warmed their hand on the fire and squeezed some milk from the breast to protect the baby from the attacks of *baobatash*. At sunset, the door of the room was kept closed. Anyone who entered into the room after sunset touched the fire and brushed her or his body with broomsticks to remove the evil wind.

The baby was never left alone during this period. At night, the birthing woman and her attendant stayed awake beside the baby. The male members in the family, especially the father, father-in-law and husband called out every now and then to keep them awake. Hamida shared a story widespread in the village,

> If the baby is left alone, a male and a female *hydor* appear as human being to steal the baby. One of them sleeps on the bed taking the baby's form. Then, the *hydor* baby develops breathing problems. Its colour changes from red to blue and later, it dies.

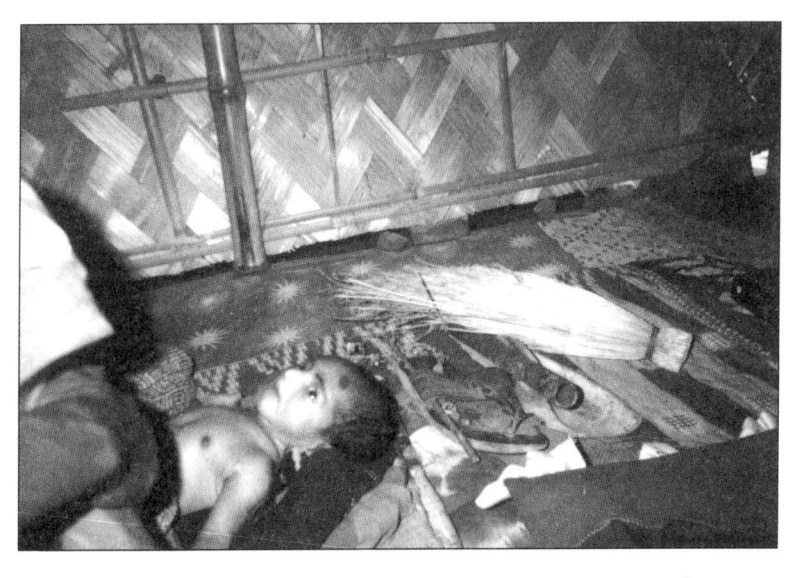

Photo 12: A baby was seen to be protected from evil spirits and evil winds by placing a broom, a leather sandal and a sickle

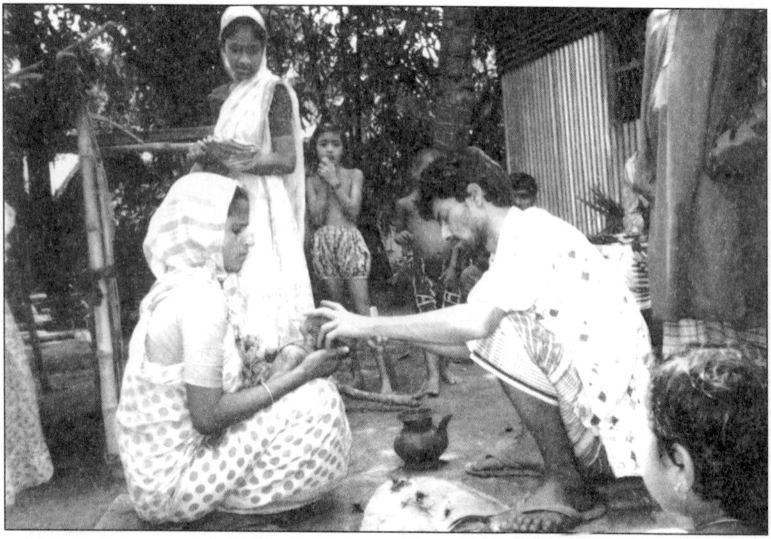

Photo 13: A barber was shaving a newborn baby's hair on the seventh day to remove pollution

Many women shared seeing a *hydor* in their dream where a deceased relative tried to snatch their baby. It was commonly known that the baby would not survive if it were given away. Concurrently, women laughed at their story about *hydor*. They also raised their concern about how the vaccine and medicine introduction gradually diminished the appearance of *baobatash* and hydor.

Strict observance of norms depended upon how the birth of baby was valued. Marsheeda said,

> When my first daughter was born, I had to follow all the *niyom-kanun* (rules and norms). After that, I gave birth to five daughters. I didn't follow anything and nothing happened to them. My last child was a boy. I had to follow *niyom-kanun*, as my mother-in-law insisted on that.

Similarly, Tohmeena strictly followed all the rules when her son was born after the birth of two girls and the death of one son. I saw Tohmeena's husband sleeping on the veranda. She said, "He comes home late and sleeps outside. He does not want to bring *hydor* inside the room." Even with the observance of rituals, she was suspicious of their success. She said, "*Apa,* I followed the same *niyom-kanun* (rules and norms) when my other son was born, but we could not keep him alive. I am following this because my *murubbis* (elders) say so. I don't know how things happen." Marium and her husband also stayed as close as possible to their only daughter after she was born. The women also told me about how male family members stayed awake throughout the first six nights in the veranda. Hamida said, "Men stay as *prohori* (watch guard) to watch whether *hydor* crosses the door. The lamps are kept lighted. They sing and keep telling stories throughout the night." These rituals were observed in accordance with the child's importance in the family.

Observance of Food Taboos

Various food taboos existed in *Apurbabari* village.[6] I noticed that the restriction of food was more vigilantly observed after childbirth. Along with many other women, Raheemon said, "I eat everything during my pregnancy." However, many women were reluctant or not allowed to eat *bhalo bhalo khabar* (very good food) during pregnancy. They believed that it would lead the fetus to grow big.[7] The very good food was synonymous with nutritious food in which they included meat, fish, egg and milk. Vitamin intake was seen to increase the size of the baby. The birthing women were discouraged to take vitamins. In one birth event at which I was present, the labour period seemed to be taking a long time. The women attended the birth were discussing about how nutritious food and vitamins made the fetus bigger. The discussion reminded me that I gave the birthing woman vitamin-B complex tablets for treating her angular stomatitis[8]. Surprisingly, the birthing woman pointed her finger to me and said, "*Apa* gave me vitamin *bori* (tablet)." I felt very embarrassed because all the women sitting there gave a suspicious look to me. On the other hand, eating rice was believed to reduce the size of the baby. Women agreed that a stomach stuffed with rice filled up the space in the abdomen and the fetus did not have room to grow bigger. The whole account suggests that in rural areas women were encouraged to eat rice but not nutritious food, like egg, milk, fish and meat in order to keep the fetal size smaller.

The food taboo was commonly observed till the sixth day of birth. Intake of meat, fish and lentils was specifically restricted. Women believed that evil spirits were very much fond of fish and meat. Eating fish and meat attracted evil spirits to nursing mothers and eventually harmed the baby. Women also believed that intake of meat, fish, egg and cold water delayed uterine involution and resulted in continued bleeding from uterus. They commented, "Your *naar* (womb) will remain *katcha* (unhealed) if you eat fish, meat and egg and drink cold water." In addition, some women believed that fish without scales was permissible to eat during the post-partum period. Hafizabibi said, "We gave non-scaly fish to my daughter-in-law. Evil spirits move with fish scales. If she eats non-scaly fish, nothing will happen to the baby." These continual discourses influenced women to abide by certain social customs.

Living with Fear of Birth and Death

Understanding of birth and death were not distinctly demarcated in rural areas. Fear of pregnancy was linked with the uncertain consequences of births. Women in *Apurbabari* associated the uncertain consequences of births with the fear of death.[9] This fear of uncertainty and death began long before birth took place. Joy of conception was there but remained together with fear of death. Like other pregnant women, Marium said, "I wonder what will happen to me. Shall I die or survive?" In fear of death, during birth event the birthing women were seen to ask forgiveness for hurting someone or committing sin. I observed Hashima asking forgiveness of Ambika, her sister-in-law, in her birth event. They both burst into tears and embraced each other. Ambika later said,

> We stopped talking to each other for a family quarrel over a goat. When I heard that she developed labour pain, I decided to visit her and resolve our silly fight. I didn't know whether she would survive. On the day of *Keyamat*[10], I will be liable to give explanation to Allah.

Hashima held similar views about the consequences of quarrel. This fear of death also brought into their mind the fear of eventual punishment given by God.

This uncertainty of survival impeded any rejoicing in the bliss of birth. Even if birth took place normally, it was not celebrated until the seventh day. Neither new clothes were stitched nor new *kanthas* (quilts) were sewn for the newly born baby. If someone sewed new quilts, they kept it hidden from the sight of pregnant women. Marium expressed her views by pointing to her newly born baby, "She is our first daughter born after two sons. We are not sure whether she will survive. What's the point of buying new clothes for her?" Without being prejudiced, like many rural women, Marium talked freely about the issue of death before her newly born daughter, but, at the same time, hesitated to dress her in new clothes. This conflicting attitude, though common, did not prevail among all women. In another instance, Tohmeena feared the death of his newly born son, but was delighted to put a new shirt on him. The significance of birth and death was hung in balance in indigenous birth.

On the other hand, scepticism about birth consequences brought physical vigour and mental strength to birthing women. It made women confront the birthing experience and conquer fear of death to procreate a new life. Raheemon said, "If I fear, I will lose my *moner shahosh* and will not be able to give birth." Women knew that they or their babies would either survive or die and the situation would worsen if fear existed. Women who gave birth alone were incessantly admired for confronting the birth single-handedly and conquering the fear of death.[11] The uncertainties returned with courage and made women encounter birth experiences fearlessly.

Personal Care

The knowledge gained from circumstances and experiences is of immense value to birthing women for personal care. In *Apurbabari* village, postpartum women usually did not use any clothes for vaginal bleeding even if their petticoats were soaked and stained with blood. Hashima said, "We don't use clothes. I change and wash my petticoats several times a day." Even in heavy bleeding, they did not wear any clothes. Rownak, born and brought up in another village said, "Once I used to use rags for my period. It's so funny. One day, my son mistakenly wiped his face with this rag. Can you imagine?" Drying stained rags openly in the courtyard was seen as a matter of *sharam*. Thus, even if some women used rags for vaginal bleeding, they dried it secretly in dark, confined places, which might eventually be a source of vaginal infections. Given that, using only a petticoat made more sense and seemed more hygienic.

Cultural knowledge influenced women to abide by certain rites. Drying *katcha naar* (the unhealed womb) was felt important to make the body *jhorjhora*[12]. Use of a hot compress by sitting on a hot brick was a common practice in this village. A brick placed near the birthing women's bed was always kept hot by warming on firewood. The birthing women sat on this hot brick to give hot compress over the mouth of birth canal to dry *katcha naar*. For the same reason, women also were seen to take a hot shower and used hot water to clean the perineal area. They stated that a hot compress reduced pain, prevented heavy bleeding and caused quick uterine involution. They also felt that if they did not continue this, *naar* (the womb) would descend, and even if, the womb did descend during childbirth, a hot compress returned it to original position. This cultural knowledge had some practical values in rural women's lives. They believed it religiously, but did not necessarily practice regularly.

Sharing and Supporting Role

The role of other women was crucial to the success of the total birthing process.[13] These women provided emotional and physical supports to birthing women. During the birth event, women shared their own stories to provide emotional support by trying to make the environment cheerful and relaxed. Kamila said, "I am telling all the stories just to keep the atmosphere lively." Most stories emerged out of their lived experiences; it could be about life or death but essentially centred on birth experiences. Women also encouraged birthing women to sustain their mental strength as labour progressed, "Please keep up your mental strength." During the course of labour, they also provided physical support while birthing women tried to adopt different postures. Massaging limbs and abdomen of the birthing women, embracing them and bringing water and food brought their emotional support. Some also cleaned the room if the birthing woman purged or passed urine or vomited. They carried out this work without complaint or any expectation. Each woman was seen to pray, "Please God, help this poor woman. Give her strength to bring the baby out." These women also recited Koranic verses to provide emotional support and reinstate birthing women's mental and physical strength.

Different rituals performed during the birth event were believed to ease and enhance the progress of labour. Apart from asking the birthing woman to walk and shake the limbs, they sat near the birthing women with their hair laid loose, and tried to collect *panipora* (sanctified water) and herbal roots. I saw one woman throwing wooden cooking spatula over the birthing hut to ease the birthing process. If the placenta was not immediately expelled, women compelled the birthing women to vomit by pushing hair into their throat[14] or by giving warm water to drink. I also observed that they put an illuminated lamp on the birthing women's head to enhance expulsion of the placenta. I came to know from a *daini* that women attending birth of a breech presentation were asked to wear *saree* upside down to change the position of the fetus.

After birth, women helped the new mother bathe in order to cleanse birth substances. They all assisted in cleaning the birthing place. Some women remained with the mother to provide assistance till the seventh day. They also helped in baby care. Before giving bath, the baby was massaged with mustard oil and left in the sun for a while, which were considered to make the baby's bones and muscles strong. After bathing, the baby was again massaged with mustard oil. Warm compression was given around the baby's umbilicus and head. These women warmed their thumb on the fire or lamp and pressed it on the abdomen around the umbilicus. They put compression on the baby's head with a cloth warmed on a lamp. Feloni said, "When a baby is born, the head becomes painful as it gets pressure on both sides. If you put warm compression on their head, it reduces pain and they sleep quietly." Women willingly shared these tasks with a birthing woman.

Role of Elder Women

The elder women included were mothers and mothers-in-law. Their role was significant in birthing women's lives throughout their pregnancy period, especially in relation to food intake and mobility. Although I heard stories from many women about how a particular mother-in-law had denied food to her daughter-in-law during pregnancy, what they shared with me and what I observed in the village did not match and reinforce village tales.

Apart from Raheemon and Shagoreen, all women I interviewed lived with their mother-in-law. Eating good food increased the size of the foetus was typical cultural knowledge circulating in the village, but none of their mothers and mothers-in-law was seen to restrict their meals. However, restriction of the movement was a common practice followed by each woman in antenatal and postnatal periods. These elder women insisted on following these particular rules and blamed birthing women if anything went wrong.

The participation of mothers and mothers-in-law in the birth event depended on how skilled and brave they were to assist in birth. In birth events of Raheemon, Shagoreen and Tohmeena, their mothers were seen to participate. Papreen's mother-in-law stayed close to her all through the event. Hashima's mother-in-law, an old woman of about 80 years continued to pray till the baby was born. Praveena's mother-in-law stayed awake throughout the night, but was not present at the birth scene. Mothers or mothers-in-law took care of birthing women during the postnatal period but it depended on their age and availability. Staying awake at night for the first six nights was an important task. Papreen's mother-in-law not only stayed awake, but also did all the chores including giving baths, washing clothes and preparing meals for Papreen.

The selection of *daini* was made consensually, but it depended on *dainis'* relationship with the family. Most *dainis* selected had attended previous births in the family. Hence, birthing women had little to say at this point and the elder women agreed to call the same family *daini*. Mothers and mothers-in-law played special role when their daughters-in-law required hospital care. Papreen's mother-in-law decided to take her daughter-in-law to the Hospital by herself, and men agreeably accompanied them. Rownak said, "I decided to go to the hospital. My mother-in-law did not say anything." Marsheeda added that her mother-in-law was very much panicked when she developed seizures and immediately accompanied her to the hospital. On the contrary, Praveena's mother-in-law was indecisive when her son wanted to take his wife to the hospital. She was frightened of hospital birth and at the same time, the *daini* strongly opposed it. Elder women played some role in decision-making, but it varied with the context.

4.2 INDIGENOUS KNOWLEDGE: THE ROLE OF *DAINIS*

Women's competence in birthing is linked with their experiential knowledge and skills (O'Neil & Kaufert, 1990). The traditional birth attendant (TBA) is a repository of indigenous knowledge of childbirth (Chawla, 2002). Yet, the presence of a TBA or *daini* in birth events is not always unambiguous. She may play a role from passive to active depending upon the situation. In some circumstances, birthing women adopt an active role, and the *dainis* may have little or nothing to do, but their mere presence adds emotional support for birthing women. Then again, *dainis'* expert interventions are felt necessary. On occasion, they manipulate their expertise resulting in aggravations of birthing problems. Even so, their knowledge, role and decisions have immense importance in a birth event. To illustrate this, I will now discuss indigenous skills and the role of *daini* as a birth attendant.

Indigenous Skills of *Dainis*

In this village, women and their families had tremendous trust in and dependence on *dainis'* knowledge and skills. One woman said, "Atiya *chachi* (aunt) does *daini's* job. She is great. Wherever she touches, it never fails." While *dainis* first started to assist in human birth, they curiously observed birth events and strove to understand women's bodily mechanisms in birthing. One Kamila said, "We don't have *pustaker gyan* (bookish knowledge). Whatever we have learnt, we learnt from observing birth events and from other *dainis*, using our own intellect." Many women began to learn this skill by assisting in birth events within the family. Some also gained this knowledge from managing deliveries of goats and cows. Yet, all of them admitted, "To be a *daini*, one should have courage." This experiential knowledge enriched their expertise and enabled them to work as a birth attendant.

Before Childbirth

Traditions of seeking care during pregnancy are rarely seen in rural Bangladesh. In recent times, pregnant women began to attend the government and NGO organised antenatal care centres. Most pregnant women I met had antenatal check-ups, yet very few willingly attended antenatal care centres.[15] The community health workers of the local NGO faced difficulties to convince women of the benefits of antenatal care. During antenatal care sessions, I observed that pregnant women looked pallid and nervous when they were examined by the field paraprofessionals. Raheemon said, "I feel scared because I don't know what she will be telling about me and my baby." Hashima added, "I don't like the way she touched my belly. She pressed so hard that I felt pain." Sitting for hours, going through the same clinical procedures, particularly abdominal examination, and listening to more or less similar comments made them disinclined to attend antenatal care sessions. In many cases, birth did not happen according to the expected date of delivery estimated by the health worker or the baby was born home safely at home even though hospital birth was strongly advised. These experiences brought distrust on newly introduced knowledge. More importantly, as pregnancy was considered as a normal phenomenon, seeking antenatal care was never prioritised.

On the other hand, the indigenous skills of *dainis* were underutilised in this domain. *Dainis* had very little role to play during the antenatal period. But, they possessed much knowledge of bodily changes occurring in this period. They confirmed pregnancy by asking women about changes in breast and abdomen. Some *dainis* were able to tell the presentation and lie of the baby by observing and touching the abdomen. In doing so, they tried to feel fetal movements. Some also established the sex of the fetus by referring to women's differential experiences:

Male baby	Female Baby
Linea Niagra[16] is as thin as a *dhaner shish*– paddy stalk	Linea Niagra is as thick as thumb
Does not move much, occasionally gives a *jhilik*	Moves constantly
Pregnant mother calling father gives birth to male baby	Pregnant mother calling mother gives birth to female
Born at 9 months	Born at 10 months
Labour pain – *kini kini betha* (little pain)	*Chara diye betha uthay* (very strong pain)

These debates among *dainis* and women did not reach a conclusion but continued endlessly. This experiential knowledge was circulating within the community from women to women.

I came to know from the field paraprofessionals that trained *dainis* were involved in identifying pregnant women and organising antenatal care centres when the TBA training programme was functioning in full swing. The strategy intended to create a relationship between the *daini* and birthing women so that their assistance would be sought during childbirth. During our conversation, the field professional explained the reasons for the discontinuation of the TBA programme. She said,

> We used to look after TBAs, trained them and involved them in identifying pregnant women and organising antenatal care centre. But, these TBAs were reluctant to work with us. They did not want to show up at antenatal sessions. They did not attend all the deliveries in the village. They were not keen to attend the refresher's training session. Besides, women do not call the trained TBAs in their birth event.

I had difficulties to locate the *daini* who received TBA training. Taljan Begum was the only trained TBA in this village and received government training many years ago in her own village. I met two trained *dainis* from the adjacent villages who were expected to perform activities in *Apurbabari* village. At present, the community health workers, who were involved in multiple activities of the NGO programme, carried out antenatal care sessions.

On rare occasions, the *dainis'* professional expertise was sought when birthing women developed pain before their expected time. *Dainis* were able to tell whether this pain was true or false. Papreen went to see a *daini* when she first developed pain. The *daini* massaged mustard oil over her abdomen and the pain gradually ceased. Labour pain would cease if it were false, and continue if it were true. Taljan, a *daini*, explained,

> I slowly massage oil over the abdomen and carefully observe the nature of pain. I allow woman to lie down for sometime. I wait to see if the pain comes back. If it does that means labour has started, and if it does not come back that means it is a false alarm.

Even though practices of antenatal care do not exist in indigenous birthing, *dainis'* expertise is used in a different manner during this period.

Progress of Labour

Rural women significantly acknowledged the skills of *dainis* in childbirth. Their knowledge and skills were seen to have considerable value in assisting women to accomplish the biological tasks of childbirth. *Dainis* judged the progress of labour by asking birthing women diverse questions. They observed the shape of the abdomen, but occasionally touched it. They examined the vaginal area with their hands, and usually did not look at the area because of *sharam*. Depending on the progress of pain, *dainis* performed varieties of tasks. They always predicted the time of delivery by observing the progress of labour and referred it to different prayer time. For instance, Feloni said, "I think, the baby will not be born before *Fazr* prayer[17] or before *Johr* prayer[18]." The *dainis* usually tried to understand the progress of labour by following the birthing women's interpretation of pain, and their feeling of fetal movement, downward thrust of fetus and pressure near anus. The progress of labour was facilitated by encouraging birthing women to empty their bladder and bowel. Taljan said, "If women evacuate the bladder and bowel, labour becomes easier for them." Birthing women followed what *dainis* suggested during delivery. This knowledge had great influence on birthing women and the female relatives.

Walking during labour pain was believed to hasten the process of labour. *Dainis* expected birthing women to walk around when pain was less strong, and encouraged them to take rest when it was very strong. Apart from it, women were asked to hold a bamboo pole or a rope hanging from the ceiling pole to push down in order to bring the baby down. If tired, birthing women were allowed to lie down or sit reclining over their female relatives. At that time, they were fanned with bamboo-made fan especially in summer, but fanning was stopped when women felt stronger pains. Feloni said, "A birthing woman will not be able to push hard if you continue to fan during her strong pains." A similar situation was also observed in the THC where the nurses and *ayahs* stopped electric ceiling fan when birthing women developed painful contractions.

Dainis did not commonly ask birthing women to bear down. A common view was, "Only a bad *daini* makes birthing women exhausted by making unnecessary bearing down." However, Papreen was given instructions to bear down when she experienced her first birth. Kamila said, "The baby will come out by itself when time arrives. We are just an *ochila*[19]." On the other hand, in Praveena's birth event, I observed that although the fetal head was stationed high, the *daini* forced her to bear down so frequently that it made her very exhausted. After five hours of struggle, she was able to give birth with severe pain and exhaustion with the assistance of another *daini*. However, among the women family members, these practices of both *dainis* were not appreciated. Thus, none of them were called in when Marium's (Praveena's aunt-in-law) birth event happened a few weeks later in the same house.

Most *dainis* did not always examine the abdomen during the actual event. When labour pain got a little strong, some touched the birthing woman's abdomen to feel fetal presentation. A few commented on the descent and engagement of the fetal head after touching the abdomen, "*Matha gaitha geche* (the head is engaged)." *Dainis* also tried to understand the fetal movement by palpating the abdomen. One *daini* stated that she tried to listen to fetal heart sound by bringing her ear close to the mother's umbilicus. She also explained,

> In one birth, the baby's leg came first. The mother told that she couldn't feel fetal movement. We knew that it was dead. But, just to check it, I pinched baby's leg. If it were alive, it would retract its leg. Right?

Not only did the birthing women act upon *dainis*' advice, but *dainis* also carefully listened to women's expressions. Hence, their knowledge and participation acted in combination to facilitate the process of birthing.

Massaging oil was an important activity of the *daini* that was believed to hasten the process of labour. The head was considered as the most respectable part of bodily organs. Thus, *dainis* put mustard oil first on the top of the birthing woman's head. Putting oil on the head was an indication of blessing birthing women to have a normal vaginal birth, to actively participate in the birth event, and to keep them in a cool temperament. The blessing was believed to be transmitted down with the oil along the locks of hair from the head of the mother to the fetus lying inside the abdomen. The subsequent massage of abdomen was done with the purpose of straightening the position of the fetus. Massaging was thought to make the position of fetus more deliverable and had both spiritual and biological implications. It not only gave a message to the birthing women, but also provided them with courage.

Shaking the waist was a common practice. A birthing woman's waist was shaken gently two to three times by holding it with both hands. A *daini* said, "This will straighten the position of the fetus and push it down." Debates continued about shaking of abdomen.[20] One medical professional told me, "*Dainis* shake the abdomen to detach the fetus from the *joraiyu* (uterus)." This view was not supported by the *dainis* of *Apurbabari* village.

Touching Birth Canal

It is widely known in Bangladesh that *dainis* frequently touch the birth passage and the fetus. Nevertheless, in *Apurbabari* village inserting hands frequently into birth canal was seen as 'something very bad' that eventually affected a *dainis*' reputation. Not only birthing women were concerned about inserting hands into the birth canal, *dainis* themselves were also reluctant to do it. One female neighbour said, "The unskilled *dainis* insert their hands frequently and make the birth canal swollen and painful. *Angtaiya ghangtaiya baccha hoyar rasta nosto koyra falai* (they damage the birth passage by too much handling)." Feloni, a *daini,* used a metaphor to explain the issue of inserting hand. She said, "The vaginal area is as soft as an eye. Inserting fingers repeatedly and carelessly causes injury to the area." Frequent handling of the birth canal drew the attention of rural women because it might eventually cause postpartum infections, vaginal and cervical injuries and birth trauma. Despite that, some women and *dainis* put stress on the importance of vaginal examination. Rownak said, "You know, sometimes *dainis* only sit, they don't even see what is happening there. If they had looked into the area and examined properly, it might have been better for mother and baby." There were opposing views about touching and not touching the birth canal, however, all agreed not to handle the birth canal frequently. Women also opposed rupturing the *panibatasha* (membrane) artificially. They became worried if the membrane ruptured before birth took place. They believed that it might aggravate the condition of the baby if labour was prolonged, and ultimately caused infections.

When *dainis* understood that the birth canal was open, they dipped their fingers into mustard oil and tried to lubricate the mouth of the vagina with oil-moistened fingers. Coconut oil was, on occasion, preferred to mustard oil, as the latter was believed to cause irritations. When pain seemed stronger, birthing women were asked to push down. Along with other women, *dainis* asked, "*Kud dey, kud dey.*" This expression means push down similar to one pushing down during defecation. However, at the same time, *dainis* employed more skills to avoid perineal tears. They guarded the perineum by firmly putting pressure over the perineal areas and anus with both great toes[21], and with clothes. On occasion, they allowed women to sit over a *piri* (wooden flat stool) to avoid perineal tears.

Dainis remained seated by holding the cord. The cord was severed and tied with thread after the expulsion of placenta. Taljan said, "If the *naar* (cord) is left loose, the placenta climbs up to the *kalija* (heart) and women will bleed to death." People believed that bleeding happened because the cord was separated from the placenta. Thus *dainis* continued to hold the cord until the placenta was expelled. After expulsion of the placenta, they tried to pull down blood from the placenta to the baby by squeezing the cord. Referring to this, one woman explained how important and useful was the expertise of a *daini*,

> In my sister's second childbirth, it happened so quickly that we did not get time to call a *daini*. The baby was born blue. It was not breathing. We thought that the baby was dead. Suddenly, the *daini* appeared. She started squeezing the cord and stroked two or three times on the baby's back. The baby started crying. If she did not have knowledge and expertise, how did she manage to bring back life to the baby?

Cord-cutting waited until the placenta was expelled[22] and the baby initiated breathing, as the placenta was believed to be the source of life.[23] If the newly babies were found in breathless state, some practices, like frying the placenta and pouring water on the umbilicus were performed to revive their lives.

In case of delayed placental expulsion *dainis* employed several methods to expel it. Apart from stimulating vomiting by pushing hair into the women's throat and giving warm water, *dainis* shared that they rubbed lower abdomen with one hand and inserted fingers along the cord and slowly pulled it out. I observed in Tohmeena's birth event that a male *dai* slowly inserted his hand along the cord to bring the placenta out. I also learnt that if the placenta was not expelled within the expected time, the cord was severed and tied around the thigh, and if women bled severely and the placenta was still retained, women were taken to the hospital.

In this village, cord-cutting and tying were considered as requiring some expertise. Thus, only *dainis* were allowed to do so. In some birth events, I was also asked to tie the cord and to check the strength of the knot. However, one woman, who had given birth in her natal village in a different area, made an interesting comment,

> I had to cut and tie the cord under the guidance of a *daini*. It is not mandatory in my natal village. But, I was told that it is good for mother and baby. *Atma* (soul or life) remains inside *naar* (cord), which binds mother with the baby.

According to her statement, only the mother possessed the authority to give soul to the baby by detaching the physical bond between the mother and the baby. More practically, the mother was taught to sever the cord because like pre-modern societies, solitary birth was still expected in some rural areas of Bangladesh.[24]

Use of stainless steel blades to sever the cord was common, but a few *dainis* still preferred to use *basher chachi* (a bamboo blade). Opposing views existed about the use of blades. Steel blades were preferred because it was iron-made and, thus, free from inflicting harms. Contrarily, *dainis* using bamboo blades believed that it was easily accessible and more importantly, free from rust whereas steel blades were sometimes rusty, which might cause *dhanustanker* (tetanus). Changing and opposing views demonstrated diversity in understandings and practices.

Emotional and Physical Supports

Someone was always needed to provide emotional and physical supports, and in most cases, it was the *daini*. Many women argued that they gave birth on their own. Nevertheless, some assistance was usually required to sever the cord, and to provide emotional and hands-on support when labour was prolonged and problems occurred. I observed that the arrival of a *daini* in a birth event enhanced emotional strength to the birthing woman and family members. Praveena eagerly waited for the *daini* who was chosen to assist in her birth event. As she lived faraway, Praveena's husband was sent to fetch her. On her arrival, Praveena and the family members seemed quite relieved. I observed that this *daini* continually made jokes, sang and shared stories to cheer up Parveena. In another instance, Shagoreen did not allow Kamila and Feloni, two *dainis*, to leave the birthing hut during the birth event. The two *dainis* sat together chewing betel leaf and telling all their stories to reduce the mother's stress. Reciting Koranic verses was commonly practised to provide emotional support. In Hashima's birth event, the *dainis* continually told her to bring back *moner shahosh* and *shoriler shakti*. The use of stories and jokes depended on the birthing woman's kin relationship with *dainis*. *Dainis* made jokes when their kin relationship with the birthing women corresponds either with grandmother or *bhabi* (elder brother's wife), but they could not make jokes if the relationship was equivalent to mother or aunt or elder sister.

Dainis were seen to provide physical support to birthing women. They changed birthing postures, gave supports at the back, massaged the body and limbs, fanned with bamboo made fan, and performed other works as well. After Raheemon's birth event, Taljan said, "I am an old woman. I don't have enough energy to give the physical support." When Hashima developed labour pain, Feloni remained awake all over the night continually accompanying her to the toilet. She also prepared the birthing place alone. *Dainis* played active roles in providing emotional and physical supports to birthing woman in order have a safer outcome.

Sometimes, but not always, *dainis* performed all the chores after the birth event was over. It depended upon whether any helping hand was available in that particular house. If no helper existed, *dainis* removed and buried the placenta, cleansed birth substances, washed clothes and smeared the floor with mud. As the placenta was associated with the life of a newly born baby, its proper burial was seen to be crucial. Placenta was usually buried in a hole dug out at the corner of a house and properly covered with earth and leaves. Inappropriate burial might attract dogs or jackals to eat placenta, which was believed to cause severe illness of newborn babies. *Dainis* were considered to perform this task very responsibly. On occasion, *dainis* were seen to live with the newly born babies and the mothers till the seventh day. In these cases, they assisted the birthing women in washing clothes, keeping the place clean, serving meals, holding the baby and more importantly, staying awake at night.

Jan Bachani Faraz

In *Apurbabari* village, *dainis* became birth attendants not out of choice or economic necessity but to meet the practical needs of birthing women. The most common response made by *dainis* was: *Jan bachani faraz* (to save life is a heavenly commandment). Even though the expression seemed very spiritual, it did not arise from supernatural calling. Kamila's experience of being *daini* happened suddenly when her sister needed the support of a birth attendant in her birth event. She shared her experience:

> At that time, I was young, newly married and didn't have my own children. It was late evening. My sister suddenly developed cramps in the stomach. She rushed to the back of the hut to empty her bowel and started screaming. No one was home. I ran after her and heard the cry of a baby. I immediately brought a knife and threads to cut and tie the cord. I have watched it before in other birth events, and managed to do it by myself. I helped clean my sister. From then on, I started to observe other *dainis'* assistance in birth event. That's how I started my *dainigiri* – practice of *daini*. I don't know how many births I have attended, and now I have stopped counting. It is someone's critical time. You can't sit around and relax. *Jan bachani faraj*. I attend the birth event not for gaining cash or kinds but to help a family. God is observing everything and will reward me for it.

This statement revealed how the situation influenced one to be a *daini*. They never linked becoming a *daini* to a spiritual inspiration. But, they believed that their devotion to saving life would bring heavenly reward. The anticipation of earning income was tangential to their main intent of being a *daini*. However, most *dainis* did not return the earthly gift given for their acts. Few *dainis* insisted on not accepting any gift because they believed that it would reduce or eliminate *sowab* (heavenly reward).

Not all women could become a *daini* if they desired to be. Becoming a *daini* was not a simple task and did not happen in a day. It was a process through which a woman experienced and learnt. Like birthing women, *dainis* also required *shahosh* (courage) and *bol* (physical strength). Momful referred to, "*Shaoshi na hoile daini hoan jai* (How could one be a *daini* if she is not brave)?" The courage and benevolent desire of helping birthing women and the practical needs led them to accept the tasks of a *daini*.

Dainis' dedication is comparable to that of *ojha* (snakebite healer). Like *ojha*, *dainis* are always available and approachable. As soon as they were summoned, without hesitation or consideration of time, place and social status, they attended the birth event to help the birthing women. Under some circumstances, they accompanied birthing women to the hospital. *Dainis*, thus, attained a respectable position among women and their families by coming forward and helping them in their life-threatening situations. I observed in a birth event that when the *daini* arrived the birthing woman was asked to touch her feet to show respect as well as to get her blessings. This was not an uncommon event when a person held a respectable position.

Professional Role

In this village, unlike *kabiraj* (herbalist), *fakir* (spiritual healer) and allopathic and homeopathy practitioners, *dainis* never existed as a profession.[25] The local healers and health practitioners practised on a regular basis, adopted it as a career and depended on it for their livelihood. On the other hand, *dainis* in this village were called upon to assist in birth because they knew *dainis' kaaj* (skills of *dainis*). These *dainis* did not depend on the income earned from their participation in childbirth. In this village, they started their activities to meet the practical needs of birthing women, but never adopted it as a career. They were considered as an experienced birth attendant holding a recognised and respectable position, but giving cash in exchange for their labour was not customary. Traditionally, local healers and health practitioners were not paid for consultations. On the other hand, spending cash for material objects, such as medicine, *tabiz* and other things was customarily practised. Surprisingly, biomedical practitioners were always paid for their consultations. As *dainis* only rendered nonmaterial services, their labour was not counted monetarily. Their payment was made in gifts depending upon each family's economic situation. The fact was that the *daini's* occupation was not established in the rural context.

In birth events, *dainis* were called upon not always for their expertise but for the nature and extent of their relationship with the family. These women lived in the village, and most came from the same socio-economic background. In certain instances, the relationship of *dainis* with the family became problematic. Kalpamoti's mother tried to avoid the *daini* who assisted her daughter's birthing, but could not. They had to call her as she was closely related to her mother-in-law. The *dainis* known as unskilled or bad *daini* were called in because of family relationships. Even if socio-economic difference existed, *dainis* from well-off families always appeared when poorer families sought their assistance. As Komolrekha's mother-in-law said, "I can't say 'no' to a poor family. We live in the same neighbourhood. We all know each other. If they face problems, don't you think we should not extend our hand?"

Dainis influenced women and the family not to seek cosmopolitan obstetric care. Their interests were not linked with pecuniary gain, but with the potential loss of communal confidence on their skills. Not only as skilled birth attendants but also as women, *dainis* strove to adhere to their own conventional expertise for the sake of their salvation, and therefore, came forward to prohibit women from seeking hospital obstetric care. I observed in Praveena's birth event that she was very exhausted after hours of struggle, but, her labour was not progressing. The *daini* being overconfident did not pay heed to anyone. Praveena's husband decided to take her to the THC. Although her mother-in-law and other women relatives were hesitant at the beginning, they subsequently agreed to transfer her to the hospital. The *daini* became angry and refused to cooperate with them. This was not an uncommon event in prolonged and obstructed labour and other pregnancy complications. *Dainis,* in fear of losing their authority of knowledge, occasionally created barriers for women and their families to seek hospital obstetric care.

A Male Dai

What drew my attention in *Apurbabari* village was the presence of a male *dai* in birth events. Moju was a male *dai* and locally known as a *shadhu* (a saint). Women did not discuss openly about Moju *dai's* involvement in their birth experience. As Rownak commented, "I was so afraid when I heard that a male *dai* would assist in my birth event. I expressed my concern to my husband. He assured me that Moju would never come if he was not requested." It was a matter of *sharam* to talk about men attending birth events. Even if he attended one's birth event, the family refused to disclose it. Moju *dai* was usually called in by his relatives. I saw him in two birth events during my fieldwork. In Tohmeena's birth event, Moju was waiting outside. He was constantly inquiring about the progress of labour. After the baby was born, the placenta was not expelled immediately. Women participating in the birth event became worried and Moju was asked to give a hand. Without looking at any women's face, he sat beside Tohmeena. Then, he held the cord with his right hand, inserted his left hand inside the birth canal, and removed the placenta without facing difficulties. While I was describing Moju's expertise to Tohmeena, she said, "Please don't tell this to my relatives and neighbours." Despite Moju's successful contribution to handling complicated cases, women considered his presence in a birth event as a matter of *sharam*.

Moju was known as an experienced, skilled *dai* in the locality. He was primarily involved in running a restaurant in the local market and also worked as a main cook in special ceremonies. I tried to communicate with him in birth events, in his house and in the restaurant, but he always avoided. His relatives said, "He feels shy." Then, I understood that he felt embarrassed to discuss his involvement in birthing. Eventually, I managed to talk to him in his house surrounded by his relatives who were extremely proud of his various skills. Moju began the task of assisting in birth events by delivering cows and goats, and gradually gained his skills by managing their complicated deliveries. He was subsequently asked to assist in human births within the family. Presently, Moju was invariably requested to attend all the complicated cases of childbirth in *Apurbabari*. I heard stories from many women how he managed breech deliveries. During my interview, I asked him how he removed Tohmeena's placenta. As Moju explained, "You can't rush. You have to know the position of the placenta. I inserted my hand and tried to find the root of the cord. I slowly pulled and it came out easily. I learnt my skills from experiences and practices." Moju was known as a skilled birth attendant and was allowed in birth events, but his presence was still not socially acceptable.

4.3 WHERE ARE MEN?

Childbirth is a women's domain. In Bangladesh, it is a socially prohibited place for men. Many cultural issues like gender, *sharam,* purdah and privacy are linked to men's exclusion from the birth event. Moreover, different understandings of bodily experiences between men and women separate out men from participating in birth events (Jordan, 1983). Although, men are physically excluded, their support is observed in many ways. At this point, men include specifically husband, father and father-in-law. I will discuss how men feel about and what role they play in indigenous childbirth.

Feeling Nowhere

Men had no physical space in a birth event in this village.[26] During the event, they did not stay within the household premises. In daylight, they all tended to attend their professional work, but at night, usually remained outside their own hut or at neighbouring houses. Men were physically secluded, but remained spiritually. Sometimes they felt redundant, as they were not able to become part of the birthing process. One said, "*Kichu korar nai* (do not have anything to do)." Their inability to feel and share experiences of childbirth made them unaware about the process of childbirth. Men, therefore, were displaced and disempowered, as birth events were dominated by women's knowledge and experiences.

Support of Men

Despite the physical exclusion of men, their spiritual presence brought them close to the event of birth. Thus, whenever some materials or persons were felt needed during birth event, it appeared or happened instantaneously. Informing the *daini,* getting things from the shop, buying medicine from the drug store and informing the barber for *choditula* were done by men. It was midnight during Shagoreen's birth event. Her husband, Abdul Haque was lying on his rickshaw van in their courtyard. I was surprised to observe that whatever items were required inside the birthing hut appeared on the veranda in a short time. Feloni, the *daini,* constantly conveyed messages to Abdul Haque, who actually waited outside for instructions. Even in the very early morning, when Abdul Haque went to his father's shop to get a stainless blade, his father was also awake. In another instance, after Raheemon's childbirth, her father bought medicine from the market without consulting Raheemon or her mother.

Tohmeena contacted me on the advice of her father-in-law. She was very emaciated and her last child died within three weeks of birth. Her father-in-law was worried about Tohmeena's physical weakness and the fate of the expected baby. This old man saw me when I accompanied Papreen to the health centre where she eventually gave birth. He asked his wife to contact me for their daughter-in-law. When I first went to their house, he anxiously wanted to know about her daughter-in-law, "How did you see my *bou* (daughter-in-law)?" I explained to him about the purpose of my research. He said, "*Ma* (mother), if you stay with my *bou*, I don't have to worry about her. Have you seen her *shashthya* (physical health)?" During Tohmeena's birthing, her father-in-law also bought homeopathic medicine that hastened the labour process. Moreover, for the first six nights after birth, he used to keep Tohmeena and her husband awake. After Papreen's son was born, her father-in-law also kept his wife awake, and told her to let Papreen sleep, "This poor girl is tired. She needs sleep." Different kinds of assistance were displayed in different settings. Men's moral and physical support was evident everywhere.

Physical Presence of Men

Men's physical presence in a birth event was unusual in *Apurbabari*. However, in certain instances, it happened when there was no helper available.[27] Shaheen's husband was obligated to remain during his wife's birth event. As Shaheen described,

> *Daini* was old. At night, she fell asleep. My husband was sitting outside. I was about to give birth. I was calling *daini*, but she was still sleeping. My husband came inside the room. I pushed down and gave birth to a baby. My husband held the baby. *Daini* woke up after hearing baby's cry.

Although physical presence of men was not acceptable in indigenous birth, Shaheen's husband had to come forward to help his wife out of necessity.

Private Encounters

All the men believed that their wife should eat nutritious foods. Unfortunately, women were not able to eat as much as required during their pregnancy. In a poor, large family, sharing meals did not leave an adequate amount of food for women. In many cases, husbands brought fruits or sweets at night for their wife when children and other family members were asleep. As Tohmeena said, "I feel like crying. How am going to eat not sharing with my children? My husband argues that I must eat because I don't get sufficient food at mealtime." On the other hand, Marsheeda was saying weepingly, "I ask my husband to buy me some bottles of vitamin, but he does not care." Yet, Marsheeda also admitted that her husband called up a doctor during her pregnancy when she was given intravenous saline, which cost them about Tk. 100 (US $ 1.60). Such interactions of men with their wives sometimes remain unnoticed.

4.4 LOCAL HEALERS AND HEALTH PRACTITIONERS

The contributions of local healers and practitioners in indigenous birthing were significant in various ways. For pregnancy ailments, poor women brought up in rural areas were accustomed to consulting with local healers (*kabiraj* and *fakirs*) in the first instance. The second choice of treatment was seeking care from local health practitioners, who practiced in the local market, but regularly visited patients in the village from door-to-door. When local health practitioners practiced in chambers, rural women sought treatment through the help of men. In this section, I will discuss the role and professional interests of healers and health practitioners.

Role of Local Healers

The professional skills of *kabiraj* (herbalist) and *fakirs* (spiritual healer) were arbitrarily differentiated. In fact, *kabiraj* treated patients with herbal medicine, and *fakir* with *tabiz* (amulets) and *panipora* (sanctified water). In my field experience, a man involved in both practices or in one was known either as *kabiraj* or *fakir*. Abdul Halem possessing only the skill of using herbal roots that enhanced labour pain was locally known as *fakir*. On the other hand, a woman practicing both practices was called as *kabiraj*. Despite women's involvement in both practices, they were not named *fakir* because only men could be *fakir* who essentially dealt with spiritual matters.

The role of *kabiraj* and *fakirs* was not insignificant during pregnancy and childbirth. They gave *tabiz* to pregnant women whose last pregnancy resulted in *moillya* (intrauterine death). It was intended for *shoril bandh* (closing the body) in order to avoid evil spells and evil winds. The advice of *kabiraj* or *fakir* was sought when labour pain became prolonged without progress. *Tabiz,* herbal roots and *panipora* were commonly given to birthing women to enhance their labour pain and to hasten the process of labour. Neonates were also given *tabiz* after the *choditula* ceremony to protect them from evil winds.

Use of herbal roots was very common among rural women during labour. Herbal root was sought from a *fakir* or a *kabiraj*. The root was tied around the left thigh of a birthing woman. As soon as the baby was delivered, it was immediately removed. It was believed that if it were not removed immediately, abdominal organs would come out through the birth canal, as the body was perceived to be a hollow tube. Abdul Halem, a village *fakir* described the rituals when collecting the roots,

> One can understand from the beginning whether that plant root works. One has to face the South and then pull the plant with the roots by keeping breathing off. If the plant comes off with the roots, it means the baby will be born without problems, but if it tears, then there will be birthing problems.

This *fakir* did not want to disclose the name of the herbs, as people in this village believed that it might damage its efficacy. However, Feloni *daini* disclosed to me in whispering voice, "You know, it is white *lajjaboti* (Mimosa plant) that is given to birthing women."

Tabiz, *panipora* and herbal roots were understood as conferring spiritual power to birthing women. In *Apurbabari*, women said that birthing women obtained physical and mental strength from the blessings of the divinity by drinking *panipora*. *Panipora* was usually sought from the *kabiraj* to accelerate the process of labour. This water was not always blessed with the Koranic *surah* (verses) recitals. In fact, the *kabiraj* read some chants from the *Sulemani ketab* (magic book of Prophet Sulaiman) and blew over the water. On occasion, local mantras were also chanted. Birthing women drank this *panipora* with deep faith. *Panipora* was also sprinkled over the head of birthing women to offer blessings. Another way of hastening labour was giving *tabiz* to birthing women. Like herbal roots, this *tabiz* was tied around the left thigh and removed as soon as the baby was delivered. Birthing women using *tabiz* for *shoril bandh* removed it once labour pain was started in order to open up the body, which was believed to remain closed with the magical charms of *tabiz*. When women and the baby became free of *napak* (pollution), both of them again were given *tabiz* to close the body in order to refrain from evil winds. Moreover, women with *shoril bandh* always avoided to come in contact birthing women to maintain the efficacy of *tabiz*.

Particular religions have very little to do with these social practices. I observed that both Islamic and non-Islamic verses were used to strengthen the power of *tabiz, panipora* and *herbal root*. Yet, performing *namaz* (Islamic prayer) was essential before preparing *tabiz* and *panipora*. Inside the shell of a *tabiz* was a piece of paper where local mantras or *Sulemani* chants were written. *Panipora* was prepared by reciting both the Koranic and non-Islamic verses and by constantly blowing over water. Even though both the male and female *kabirajes* were strong believers of Islam, their professional knowledge was not at all influenced by their own religiosity. The faith of village women and men in these practices was not affected by their religions. An educated woman in *Apurbabari* sought amulets from a Hindu *Kabiraj* to protect the baby from the evil spirits and evil winds. Her son was born with congenital defects of his fingers. This Hindu *kabiraj* tied amulets around both the baby's legs to close his body. In addition, he also closed their house *(baribandh)* by burying sacred amulets around it. This woman was embarrassed when I inquired about *baribandh* and *shorilbandh*. She said, "Listen, I don't believe in this. My mother is a traditional woman. She called the *kabiraj* to do all this in order to protect her grandson."

Professional Interests of Local Healers

The profession of *kabirajes* and *fakirs* mostly ran in the family for generations. Yet, some adopted it out of economic necessity. The local knowledge of healing was usually circulated from one generation to the next in successions. *Kabiraj* Abdul Lokman said, "I learnt this practice from my father and grandfather and from reading books. I collected many old books. I would like to pass on my knowledge to someone else regardless of sex." On the other hand, economic necessity compelled Alemon Begum to accept this profession about 50 years ago. She learnt this knowledge from a *Garo*[28] *kabiraj*,

> I became a widow with five sons and two daughters. Who will look after my family? I followed this *kabiraj* everywhere and observed his work. At the beginning, he was reluctant to teach me. Seeing my desperation, he agreed. I usually treat women and children. But, if men come, I also treat them.

She was slowly passing her knowledge on to her daughter-in-law, as her age increased. It was known in *Apurbabari* that this knowledge could only be transmitted to a person who belonged to the astrological sign of Libra.

Money earned from giving *panipora*, *tabiz* and herbal roots was not huge. Demanding money was completely prohibited in the practices of *fakir*, yet all of them earned some out of their practice. Abdul Lokman did not depend only on his practices. He was a small farmer, but seriously took his *kabiraji* profession. He showed me all the books he collected during 25 years of his profession. He said, "I try to help people. If we demand money, we will lose our spiritual power." While I was talking to him, a man came complaining about some *tabizes*, "The *tabiz* you have given for *baribandh* (closing house) is not working. My brother is behaving crazily and talking incoherently again. We have already paid you Tk. 300. What will you do now?" *Kabiraj* Lokman inquired about how the *tabizes* were buried in their house and found out faults. He went to see the man immediately. I also accompanied him. It was evening and dark in the village. On our arrival, everyone came out of the huts. The man was standing on the veranda. *Kabiraj* Lokman started chanting by placing his hand over the man's head and blew air on it. The man suddenly got his sense back and started to talk normally. *Kabiraj* asked him about the spirit, but he was not able to say anything. Then, Lokman instructed his brothers how the *tabizes* should be buried. The family members admitted their mistakes. When they wanted to pay him, he did not accept money.

Alemon Begum encountered much hardship and used to depend completely on these earnings when her children were young. She said, "I never demand money. When people pay me happily, I accept it. As my sons look after me now, I don't need money anymore." Abdul Halem who only gave herbal roots to birthing women did not accept money. He said, "You can't accept money only for this." Rural women who sought herbal roots were his close relatives and neighbours.

Both Alemon Begum and Abdul Lokman admitted that they never tried to impose professional interests on their clients. However, their views of sending birthing women to the hospital revealed different perspectives. Abdul Lokman expressed his concern, "I never restrict women to stick to *panipora* and *tabiz* only. If labour does not progress within certain time, I ask the family to take the birthing woman to the hospital." Alemon Begum also did not get involved in treating serious pregnancy complications, but she ridiculed women for going to the hospital, "Women are changing. They are losing trust on *kabiraji* medicine. If something little happens, birthing women are taken straight to the hospital. Seeking care from the hospital is a *juger chol* (current fashion of a new era)." The differing views about birthing problems were perhaps related to generational change and professional interests. Abdul Lokman coming from a new generation did not rely only on his practice, which was contrary to the circumstances of Alemon Begum.

Role of Local Health Practitioners

In *Apurbabari* village, local health practitioners practised both homeopathic and allopathic medicine. Their role in pregnancy and childbirth was not prominent. Depending upon their familiarity and accessibility, local practitioner's advice was occasionally sought during pregnancy. Pregnant women's husbands usually served as the go-between to discuss their wives' ailments with the local health practitioners. The health practitioners usually prescribed homeopathic medicine for pregnant women, as it was believed to cause less or no side-effects. Believing in hot and cold notions, rural women preferred homeopathic medicine during pregnancy. They not only considered it as a cold medicine but also believed that it had no side effects. Administering intravenous saline during the antenatal period was not uncommon. I was with a health practitioner in *Apurbabari* while he administered intravenous saline to a pregnant woman. Women felt proud to receive intravenous saline and described how this 'magic medicine' brought their physical energy back.

During labour, use of both homeopathic and allopathic therapy was observed. At the beginning of labour, if pain was slight, the local practitioners prescribed homeopathic medicine to enhance pain and dilatation of cervix. They gradually increased the dosage of medicine after thoroughly inquiring about the progress of labour. On occasion, they also used allopathic treatment. When the labour process became prolonged, the poor family requested them to continue treatment at home in order to avoid hospital birth. In that case, the local health practitioners consulted with *dainis* about the progress of labour, as men were not allowed to examine the vaginal area. After consultations, they administered oxytocic drug[29] in intravenous saline to birthing women. This treatment sometimes succeeded. If not, they suggested that the family take the birthing woman to hospital. In the postpartum period, allopathic analgesic and ergot drugs were prescribed for birthing woman to reduce their pain and vaginal bleeding. Commonly prescribed analgesics were diclofenac and ergots were ergometrine. Sometimes, intravenous saline was administered to bring back physical energy to birthing women. Homeopathy was hardly used in the postpartum period, but was largely prescribed for treating neonatal illness.

Professional Interests of Local Health Practitioners

In *Apurbabari,* the profession of local health practitioners was mostly linked to their fathers' association with medical profession. Sharup Bakshi's father was a homeopathy doctor in their village. In spite of his willingness to obtain MBBS degree, he failed to get admission into the Medical College. This led him to study for a degree at a Homeopathy College and to undertake government paramedic (medical assistant) courses. He had many patients in adjacent villages. In the morning, he rode on his bike to visit patients in their houses. In the afternoon, he consulted in his chamber-cum-drugstore attached to his house. This was located in the thana town and two kilometers away from *Apurbabari* village.

Mahbubur Rahman was also a local health practitioner. Despite the fact that he had a master's degree from the Islamic Madrasah University, he did not pursue long-course training in homeopathic or allopathic treatment. He received short training to qualify as a rural medical practitioner (RMP). Like Sharup Bakshi he also visited patients in their villages. However, Mahbubur Rahman was mostly seen in his chamber located in the local market, where both homeopathic and allopathic medicines were sold. Attached to the chamber was his tailoring shop where he also made dresses along with his *karmocharis* (paid workers). As his chamber was located close to *Apurbabari,* the village men mostly consulted him and bought medicines from his store.

The professional interests of local practitioners in birthing care were linked to their income earning and reputation. They did not charge consultation fees when attending patients, but they mostly sold medicines at high prices. The poor villagers did not object to it, as they were allowed to make payments in instalments with no interest. Abdul Jaber, a village man said, "*Apa*, it is a great relief to us. We can't afford to pay the total amount of money immediately. If local doctors were not here, I don't know what we would have done." In this context, Mahbubur Rahman said,

> This practice has been going on for generations. We can't change it. Besides, we know all of them. How do we ask money for consultation? They are poor. They can't give money all at a time. But, they always pay it off.

The flexible payment system also made poor, rural families to seek care from local health practitioners.

Village people had tremendous respect for them. The local practitioners spoke the local language, entered into the house and called women as *bhabi* (sister-in-law) or *chachi* (aunt) depending on their age. I saw Sharup Kumar Bakshi sitting with a woman in the courtyard and listening to her problems. A few other women also sat and discussed this woman's problem to him. He listened to the women patiently. During birth event their consultation with *daini* brought them close to birthing women and made them understood the progress of labour. Sharup told me, "Yes, Sharnarupa *daini* knows a lot. She assisted my wife and sister during their birth experiences, and constantly reported their progress of labour." Constant and close interactions with rural women at their own home made the local health practitioners more approachable.

4.5 SUMMARY AND CONCLUSION

In exploring indigenous birth practices, core issues were identified from multiple perspectives including my own observational experiences. In this study, women's knowledge was expressed in their understanding of birth, and feeling of *moner shahosh and shoriler shakti* and bodily experiences during childbirth. This knowledge allowed women to decide the extent of their involvement in the birth experience. Maintaining silence before and during birth was identified as an important issue that was related to their notions of *sharam*. In the birth event, the role of other women became visible in providing physical and emotional support to birthing women. More crucial was the participation of the *daini* in birth event. In accomplishing birth, not only did they apply their skills, but their involvement became also significant with providing emotional, psychological and physical support to birthing women. Sharing of knowledge and experiences during the event facilitated the process of birth and eased the situation.

An unusual observation was the existence of a male *dai* whose assistance was sought specifically in complicated births, but he was not able to be part of the event, as the presence of a man was considered to be a matter of *sharam*. Men were not directly involved in the birth event, but their participation was displayed in providing physical support from outside. The involvement of the husband was identified in one particular birth event when the wife needed urgent assistance.

Commemorating birth was a communal event, but understandings of pollution and evil spirits and winds resulted in birthing women and their babies being confined for the first six nights. Women also followed rules and restrictions related to food intake and mobility. On the seventh day, ceremonial rituals cleansed women and babies from pollution and freed them from confinement.

Different groups of people were involved in providing care to birthing women. The local healers and health practitioners had some role in providing amulets, sanctified water and herbal roots to birthing women. These were used in the context of local, cultural understandings of the body associated with supernatural forces. The local health practitioners treated birthing women either with homeopathic or allopathic treatment. Local healers and health practitioners had shared cultural knowledge with rural women that made them more approachable. The construction of indigenous birth was seen to be embedded not only in the participation of birthing women, but also in the participation of multiple players whose social, professional and political interests were visible.

In the following chapter, I will describe cosmopolitan obstetric practices from the perspectives of women, doctors, nurses, hospital administrators, hospital staff, special *ayahs*, patient's attendants and many others that unravel scenarios of hospitals.

Notes

[1] In some African societies, birthing women are usually assisted by older female relatives only in the first birth. The cultural ideal of giving birth alone is achieved after the first birth (Biesele, 1997).

[2] Sweets are distributed in Bangladesh after the birth of a baby usually among well off people.

[3] In many other societies, the cultural expression of pain and tolerance means facing childbirth bravely. This brings pride and honour to birthing women (Biesele, 1997; Sargent, 1989. Shostak, 1981)

[4] Gardner remarked in her anthropological research in rural Bangladesh that birthing women are seen as dangerously polluted (Gardner, 1991).

[5] People coming in contact with *chochi* women were also regarded as *chochi* and vulnerable to attacks of malevolent spirits (Rozario & Samuel, 2002).

[6] In many other places of Bangladesh, various taboos of food exist (Goodburn, et al., 1994; Goodburn, Gazi & Chowdhury, 1995; Blanchet, 1984).

7   In many traditional communities of India, restrictions of foods are observed for not allowing the growth of fetus (Gupta, et al., 1997).

8   Angular stomatitis is an ulcer at the angle of mouth occurred due to Vitamin B-6 deficiency.

9   An African study also found in Ju/'hoan society the fear of death and challenges related to birth event (Biesele, 1997).

10 In Islamic faith, Keyamat is the day of final judgment.

11 In many pre-modern cultures, women are praised for participating in solitary birth (Biesele, 1997; O'Neil & Kauffert, 1990; Sargent, 1989).

12 The literal translation of *jhorjhora* is refreshed and free from morbidity (Biswas, Dasgupta & Sengupta, 1968).

13 According to Jordan (1983), participation of others is an integral part of birth event providing human companionship and emotional supports. Women become much more involved because of their bodily co-participation and co-experience with birthing women.

14 Triggering vomiting is an identical practice suggested by Kitzinger (1991) that propels the placenta down.

15 Other research documented similar observations (Afsana & Mahmud, 1998; Chowdhury, Mahboob & Chowdhury, 2002).

16 Lina Niagra is a pigmented line developed during pregnancy period, which extends from umbilicus down to public symphysis.

17 Among Muslims, it is a morning prayer that occurs before sunrise.

18 Among Muslims, it is a prayer that occurs at noon.

19 *Ochila* is a common word used in rural Bangladesh. It means ' through which a work is accomplished.'

20 In many other societies, shaking is also observed to make the fetus loose (Kay, 1982).

21 Similar observation is seen in birth practices of Sierra Leone (MacCormack, 1982)

22 In Guatemala, cord is cut after expulsion of placenta (Cosminsky, 1982)

23 In other part of Bangladesh, the cord was not severed before placental expulsion and initiation of baby's breathing because placenta is believed to be a source of life (Blanchet, 1984).

24 In African pre-modern societies, the mother is taught to sever the cord because they prefer to have solitary birth in a bush (Biesele, 1997), whereas in Bangladeshi literature, cutting cord is linked with dangerous pollution, thus birthing women is likely to do it (Blanchet, 1984; Rozario, 1998, 2002).

25 In Latin America and Africa, practice of TBA is considered as a profession.

26 In many different cultures, husbands are included in the birth event (Jordan, 1983)
27 Men were allowed in birth event when no assistance was found (Rozario, 1998).
28 *Garo* is a tribe living mostly in hilly areas in the Northern part of Bangladesh.
29 Drugs used in biomedicine to enhance uterine contractions

Chapter 5
Cosmopolitan Obstetrics: Construction of Birth in Hospitals

Birth is defined and redefined by people participating in it no matter where it occurs. I never seriously thought about how hospital obstetric services were organised for poor, rural women when I was an intern resident in a teaching hospital between 1983 and 1984. Yet, some events and experiences from this period still left an imprint in my mind. Later, in my academic life, I began to explore literature on hospital obstetric practices (Davis Floyd, 1992; Jordan, 1983; Martin, 1989; Oakley, 1980). Even then, I did not fully realise or anticipate the consequential experiences until I started my own research in this arena. I have gained deeper understanding of hospital birth practices during my fieldwork than I was ever able to visualise as an intern or a practicing doctor. More I get acquainted with it more I understand the role of multiple players in constructing hospital birth practices.

The purpose of this section is to offer thematic representations of birth experiences, which are multi-voiced, multi-dialogic contributing to the construction of birth in the hospital. In this chapter, I address women's experiences of hospital birth, my own experiences, and the roles of different individuals affecting women's hospital-based, obstetric care. At the outset, I shall elaborate my immediate experiences in the hospital, which is followed by women's birth experiences. Voices of doctors, nurses, patient-attendants, *ayahs* and others will reinforce the state of cosmopolitan obstetric care in Bangladesh. At the end, I will discuss the role of fieldworkers in providing pregnancy-related care in *Apurbabari* village. In this chapter, although I describe events from THC, my discussion of hospital care refers mainly to practices carried out in the Medical College Hospital because the former does not manage complicated pregnancies and the duration of hospital stay is very short not exceeding more than 24 hours for uncomplicated vaginal delivery.

5.1 EMBODIED FEELING OF BEING A DOCTOR

Becoming a doctor means entry into a prestigious position in an elitist milieu. With the exception of a clergy, this is the only profession where a person is addressed with an honourary title, such as Doctor in everyday language, which has a profound effect on one's self-image (Wagner, 1997). Wearing a white apron[1] makes physicians feel different from others and signals a superior status. This experience becomes embodied and engenders a feeling of an authority in their everyday life. I consciously tried to excise the title from my name, but it is difficult to do so. The advantages of using the title are countless. I could not avoid it while I sought permission for my fieldwork in the hospital, otherwise I would have had to go through complex bureaucratic procedures. As a doctor I was easily accepted into the professional group, which has strong solidarity and a shared, privileged position. But, I never felt a sense of ownership to this group. My sense of being a doctor never existed. Shall I be considered a traitor if I defy the power and politics of cosmopolitan obstetrics through my research?[2]

5.2 MEETING DOCTORS IN THE HOSPITAL

My first interactions with doctors in the Medical College Hospital happened during an academic discussion on maternal health. The entire discussion revealed their absolute trust in the scientific knowledge of cosmopolitan obstetrics. It was an in-house seminar on recurrent abortion (miscarriage). The presentation was made about a 27 year-old woman who had a history of one stillbirth and seven repeated abortions. During her ninth gravidity, she was admitted into the Obstetric Unit of the hospital and treated till the baby was born. The obstetricians were excited about the success of their treatment. The woman was provided with good obstetric care. Her cervix was stitched with some MacDonald's suture. Issues were raised about the introduction of new and sophisticated treatment for cervical incompetence, and the pros and cons of different surgical treatment. Surprisingly, the discussion neither considered the woman's previous birth experience in the village nor addressed the practices of TBAs and the issues of community care. I tried to open up discussion with the doctors about the TBAs role in the community. However, my concerns went unheeded. Their interests centred on the sophisticated treatment procedures and the importance of cosmopolitan obstetric care.

5.3 MY IMMEDIATE EXPERIENCES IN THE HOSPITAL

On entering the hospitals especially the Medical College Hospital, I observed some events that remained as first-hand experiences. When I worked as a medical doctor in the hospital, I observed the events, but did not dwell on them, simply considering as part of everyday life. At this point, I will begin with my immediate experiences in hospitals.

Too Many People

The first experience after entering the hospital was the *jonotar michil* (mass of people) I met. I was very much saddened by the sight of people in hospitals. I was brought-up and lived in this country for most of my life surrounded by millions of people, but, why was I overwhelmed with sadness? This question is, particularly, pertinent because I was mentally depressed to observe the sparse number of people when I first went to Ottawa, Canada with my husband[3] and son in 1985. I used to sit by our apartment window, and sudden glimpses of one or two bystanders on the street brought a smile to my face. When I came to Perth, Australia to study for my PhD these feelings returned as the plane was landing. I was able to capture glimpses of Perth. Memories of Canada came back because Perth is also an identical place barren of people. When the sparse number of people in Canada and Australia dispirited me, then, why did I become sad at seeing the flood[4] of people in the hospitals of Bangladesh? The fixed beds were all occupied, and extra beds were placed on the floor in between the fixed beds. Patient's attendants were sitting here and there. The verandas, corridors and the outpatient department all were packed with people moving with desperation. The antenatal and postnatal wards in Obstetric Units had fixed beds for 72 patients, but received two to three-folds patients everyday. More patients were observed in the antenatal examination room, labour room and eclampsia room[5] too. The total capacity of this hospital building was 500, but each day the number of patients exceeded 1200. More importantly, three to four persons accompanied each patient that created a crowded, chaotic environment in the hospital.

Unclean Environment

My second immediate impression was the unclean, hospital environment. While I walked carefully to avoid rubbish on the dry hospital floor, the rural women walked in a relaxed manner on the wet, dirty floor. It was the weekly cleansing day in the hospital. Three special *ayahs* were engaged in washing the hospital floor in the Obstetric unit, but only with water. It took about two hours to wash the long corridor passing between the antenatal ward and the operating theatre. Muddy water splattering on the floor stopped me from walking over it. I had to stop until it became slightly dry. Rural women and their attendants continually crossed the wet, muddy floor without showing any repugnance.

Although regular mopping was carried out, the antenatal ward, labour room, eclampsia room, postnatal wards and corridors remained dirty. The floor became discoloured sticky with dirt, and speckled with sputum, blood, vomitus and urine in some places. Pieces of foodstuff, cottons and papers were scattered on the floor. The tin bowls used as rubbish bins were left open under the bed emitting foul smells. Bed linen looked discoloured and old being changed only when new patients arrived. The windows were mostly closed creating a suffocating atmosphere. Patients, attendants, *ayahs* and even nurses threw water on the floor and wall while cleaning their hands or rinsing their mouth. People also spat on the floor and walls. When I enquired why a patient did not spit into the tin bowl, she said, "How can people spit over and over at the same place? The sight of my own spit on the *gamla* (bowl) nauseates me." The outside drains were all open and filled with plastic bags and rubbish. The open garbage bins on the veranda were filled with sand. Persons walking by threw rubbish and spat into it.

I tried to experience the hospital toilet, but failed. It was wet, smelly and full of dirty cottons. "Please do not throw sanitary napkins everywhere. Throw it in the garbage bin" stated the notice in front of the toilet. A garbage bin was placed opposite to this toilet. The foul air of the toilet circulated inside the wards and made the atmosphere unbreathable. Because of this stench, working inside the wards was sometimes difficult. A doctor proudly said, "We live in filth and work with filth." However, she did not question herself how this filthy atmosphere led to hospital infections.

When I returned to the village after my first visit to the hospital, Rownak's first question was, "*Apa*, did you visit the toilets in the hospital?" She continued, "I still can't forget my experience in the toilet. It was so smelly. The floor was flooded with urine and water.

I went in and my half legs were dipped into dirty water." The nurse-in-charge later told me, "The cleaners clean the toilets everyday. But, people do not know how to use a toilet. They throw water everywhere. They urinate on the floor instead of sitting on the toilet pan." In response to my question, a patient said, "Who will sit on the toilet pan for passing urine? People defecate, but do not flush with water. It's dirty." A cleaner in the THC raised her problem, "How will you keep the toilet clean? Is it always possible to fetch water from the ground floor? We haven't had a water supply for more than five months." All these factors exacerbated the situation resulting in unclean toilets.

When I talked to the ward master, he took me around the hospital showing the nine, cement-made garbage disposal tubs built in different places. He explained how rubbish was collected and taken by the municipal truck, and the difficulties of maintaining cleanliness. He said,

> In each ward, there is one toilet per 24 patients. Now, the number of patients is increased two to three fold. With each patient you will see five attendants. At night, people sleep on the veranda. Where will they go to the toilet? For four to five months, we do have not had a supply of phenyl or bleaching powder. People throw rubbish everywhere. There is no specific place to throw rubbish. We try hard to keep it all clean.

Despite efforts to keep the hospital clean, the environment was terribly unhygienic. While I was walking through the hospital with the ward master, I asked myself how we all were surviving here.

5.4 EXPERIENCING HOSPITAL: WOMEN AND THEIR FAMILIES

Rural women and their families underwent diverse experiences while attending hospitals. Decision making was delayed due to their fear of hospital. After arrival at hospital, women and their families encountered many different people and had various experiences in an entire alien environment. It is the essence of this experience, which I explore in this section.

Beginning Journey to the Hospital

In the village, before starting for the hospital, women feared to face an unknown environment and unfamiliar faces, meet uncaring doctors and nurses, experience surgery, and encounter impending hospital expenditures. These pre-conceived fears delayed the process of decision-making. On the other hand, Rownak explained, "To get good services in the hospital, you need to know someone there. If you don't know anyone, you are in trouble." Shaheena, a schoolteacher, expressed similar views about the hospital. In *Apurbabari* when Praveena had prolonged labour pain, her husband became worried, but was hesitant to take her to the THC. He expressed his concern, "We did not go to this hospital before. We don't know the place. What will happen if the doctor and nurse do not turn up?" Her mother-in-law was concerned about the methods employed in hospital delivery, particularly surgical treatment. She said,

> I have heard that in the hospital they insert their whole hand into the birth canal by covering it with a *haat moja* (gloves). They also unnecessarily cut their birth canal. I am afraid of taking her to the hospital.

Decision to seek hospital care in time was delayed or postponed or stopped due to such apprehensions. Praveena's baby was eventually born at home despite her severe painful birthing experience.

Finding an appropriate person to accompany the woman and family to the hospital, to give them directions and to communicate with hospital staff was very important. Everyone looked for a person who was familiar with the hospital environment. In *Apurbabari* village, Monira and Momful were usually chosen to accompany villagers to any hospital or clinic for a simple matter. Papreen's mother-in-law was sad when they were not able to convince Monira to accompany them to the THC during Papreen's first childbirth experience. She said, "We must convince Monira to go with us. We don't know anything in the hospital. Doctors and nurses will be annoyed if we can't communicate with them." They finally persuaded Monira to accompany them.

Village women not only feared surgical treatment, but were also highly critical of male doctors seeing their bodies. All the women I met asked me, "Why do doctors cut the vaginal area during childbirth?" I could not give them a satisfactory answer. Rahena was reluctant to go to the THC and stated, "I did not want to go to the hospital. I knew, they would cut my vaginal area and they did." Her fear became real. She was given an episiotomy incision during her first childbirth experience in the THC. Having an episiotomy incision was considered a social stigma, 'a mutilated body'. Anowara explained to me, "Body parts have become defective on cutting vaginal area. It also affects the sexual relationship with the husband[6]." These concerns made women hesitant to seek hospital obstetric care.

The rural women from this village were worried about the presence of male doctors in hospital birth. In the THC, where I did fieldwork, the appearance of male doctors during childbirth was quite unusual, whereas, their access to Obstetric Unit was quite common in the Medical College Hospital. It was not that male doctors were sensitive to cultural issues in the THC, but not in the Medical College Hospital. In both places, the reasons for the presence of male doctors were associated with their professional roles and responsibilities and the existing hospital practices. Rural women linked the presence of male doctors with the issue of *sharam*. Sharoma said,

> I don't dare to go to the hospital. *Purush* (male) doctors work there. They will see your body. It's a matter of *sharam*. Everyone in the village will know that a *purush* doctor has seen your body. They will tease you and also insult you.

All the women I interviewed were concerned with the violation of their privacy by the presence of male doctors in birth events.

Immediate need for a large sum of money put the poor villagers under tremendous pressure. They collected some cash before their arrival at the hospital, but had no idea about the amount of money required for hospital treatment. In my observation, when Papreen was going to the THC, her father-in-law sat with the male relatives and neighbours in the courtyard to have a meeting. I became worried and asked Saleha, Papreen's aunt-in-law, "You are being late. We should start immediately." She said, "We don't have money. The men are deciding how much money will be needed and how the money will be collected." Papreen's father-in-law borrowed some money from a relative and sent Papreen's husband to the local market to collect more money. The process of collecting money considerably delayed their departure for the THC.

Moving Hither And Thither

Running all over the place was a common problem faced by women at different points in their journey from home to hospital. In my observation, the first disappointment faced by the family was the refusal of treatment at the THC from where they were referred to the Medical College Hospital. Romila stated, "The small hospital couldn't treat my problem and sent me here to the big hospital. We ran here and there." Before reaching the Medical College Hospital, they had to change transports several times. Romila's husband said,

> We took the rickshaw to go to the Thana hospital. Later on, they sent us to the district hospital. We took a bus to reach there. They also couldn't treat my wife's problem. From there we hired an ambulance to come to this big hospital.

Rownak also shared her experiences about reaching the hospital,

> We went to the Thana hospital on my brother's-in-law rickshaw van. From there, my husband took me to the bus station on a rickshaw. We arrived in town by bus and hired a rickshaw to reach the doctor's chamber and afterwards came to the hospital.

Denial of treatment in different health facilities forced families to move from place to place. When they eventually arrived at the tertiary hospital more incidents and experiences awaited them.

In the emergency room, rural women and their families began to face trouble during their admission to the Medical College Hospital, and continued to encounter difficulties until their discharge. From the emergency room, the admitted pregnant women were brought to the antenatal check-up room, moved either to labour room or operating theatre or antenatal ward and were subsequently sent to the postnatal ward. For laboratory tests, they were taken to different places within the hospital campus. The statement of Rownak where she narrated moving all over the place was associated with hassles at different places and situations. She said,

> If you go to the hospital, you have to run here and there (*dour paron lagey*). When my children were born at home, I just stayed in and nobody knew about it. But, when I needed hospital care for my second pregnancy, the whole village came to know about it and many people accompanied me. In the hospital, we don't know anything. We can't read and write. We run here and there. For running, you need someone who went to the hospital before. For reading you need someone who can read. Who has so much time to accompany and who has so much money to bear the costs? I hate moving around. Not only you run here and there, you face loads of unknown people before you come back home. Isn't it *sharam* for a woman?

The experience of running from pillar to post not only caused physical and emotional exhaustion, but it also affected their cultural emotion, that is, *sharam*. Having a rural background with no reading and writing skills made birthing women disempowered in the hospital, and hence, humiliated and betrayed at every point. Subsequently, they returned to the village overtired and with bitter experiences of losing dignity and privacy.

Getting Admission into the Hospital

In the emergency room, the duty doctor admitted all the women coming with obstetric problems into the hospital. They wrote a short note on the patient's file without directly communicating with the women. During admission, each patient was charged slightly over the standard fee. In front of this room, it was clearly written: Admission fee is Tk 7.50. However, paying Tk 10 instead of Tk 7.50 for the hospital admission seemed acceptable to each patient and their attendants.

The first surprise began when women and their families faced bargaining with special *ayahs* and ward boys. The special *ayahs* awaited new patients in the long corridor adjacent to the emergency room. As soon as the patients were admitted they came forward for assistance. Patients coming from rural areas sought the *ayahs*' assistance, as they were not able to locate anything in the hospital. Both ward boys and special *ayahs* pushed the trolley carrying the patient to the antenatal examination room. The problems arose when they demanded cash for their task. The patient and their companions did not anticipate paying the ward boys who were paid hospital staff and special *ayahs*, who they thought to be hospital staff, for such a petty task. The patient's companions started to bargain, and the ward boys and *ayahs* became annoyed. Shahana's mother said, "I told them, we are poor. We can't pay the amount you ask, but we won't make you unhappy." Even if they could not make the payment immediately, they gave money afterwards.

I heard the stories from patients, nurses and *ayahs* about hospital *dalals* (agents or touts) abducting patients to private clinics before their admission into the hospital. During my fieldwork, I was not able to observe such a scene near the emergency room. However, I met two *dalals* in the outpatient department. It was not actually kidnapping, but patients were abducted from the hospital to the private clinics where doctors did private practice. Those abductors were locally known as *dalal*. The two *dalals* I met introduced themselves as a hospital representative. One of them said,

> I come here almost every day looking for a patient. Many patients come to see an obstetrician and aren't sure where they should go. We convince them to go to the clinic. Besides, doctors refer patients to the clinic. We also arrange for those doctors to perform operations on that particular patient.

He tried to illustrate the better quality and the lower cost of clinic services compared to those of the hospital. A nurse spoke of her friend how she was cheated and taken to a private clinic by a nursing hostel's security guard. However, they were not able to do anything, as the security guard denied the whole fact. Most *dalals* worked in private clinics and some also in the hospital. This business made some additional income for them.

Feeling Lost in the Hospital

Village people, at present, were not unaware of large buildings due to their exposure to cities and mass media as well. But, physically entering and walking in the hospital building was a different experience. Shahana's case was a perfect example. Her mother and mother-in-law were scared to death in hospital buildings. When the doctor instructed them to buy medicine, they embraced each other and started crying. In fear of getting lost, they were hesitant to leave each other. Her mother said, "We were terrified by the massiveness of the building. It's like a puzzle. One can easily get lost. We feared losing contact with each other." The mammoth structure of the buildings did not bear any resemblance to buildings in their customary environment. Besides, the rooms were scattered all over the places. As most did not have any education, finding the specific place by following written instructions was not easy for them. As a result, the village people were always seen moving around the hospital in a small group.

Women Remaining Silent

I observed a great difference between Papreen's behaviour during her birthing experience at home and at the hospital. Papreen, a young woman of 18 conceived for the first time. Her aunt told me, "Papreen is having labour pain for more than three days. She is not cooperating, not pushing and not letting anyone touch her vaginal area. She is yelling at us – her mother-in-law, *daini* and me." I entered into the hut. She was lying on the floor moaning with pain. As soon as she saw me, she became quiet. The family decided to take her to the hospital. When we arrived at the local health complex, Papreen's behaviour suddenly changed. She became very quiet and accommodating. The nurse examined Papreen and immediately started saline and oxytocin. She did not communicate verbally with Papreen. The female attendants responded to her inquiries. The nurse inserted her gloved hand into the vagina consistently stretching the vaginal walls. Within an hour, the baby was born. Papreen later shared with me, "I was very scared. I had so much pain, but didn't utter a word. I wanted to be quiet. I didn't know what they would do to me or to my baby."

Participating in Own Birth Experience

In the hospital, the birthing women were not allowed to participate fully in their own birth experiences. My observation in the labour room revealed how women's birth experiences were regulated and controlled by the biomedical professionals. Rumpa was not allowed to move. Her two hands were strapped down. Oxytocin in intravenous saline was being administered. An antibiotic injection was also given. She was catheterised with an intra-urethral catheter to relieve urine. An intern doctor gave her instructions to bear down, "Push, push." She also took preparations for giving an episiotomy incision. Rumpa was not informed about the incision on her perineal area. Her perineum was bulging. The intern doctor with her unskilled hands gave an episiotomy incision on her perineal area. It started to bleed. The doctor seemed a bit nervous. She instructed Rumpa to push down. The baby was born after several pushes. After severing the cord, the doctor took the baby for resuscitation. As the baby seemed normal, she came back to Rumpa. By then, the placenta was expelled. After stitching the episiotomy incisions, the intern doctor started to fill in the patient's record by taking history from a special *ayah* who in turn asked questions to Rumpa and her mother.

In this medical mode, the birthing woman's experience started with physical confinement to a labour table that went against her will. Rumpa expressed her aversions, "It is strange! One can't choose to stand or sit in the labour room or even move on the labour table." Rumpa's verbal consent was neither taken nor was she informed of what was being done to her body. The interactions between the doctor and the woman did not involve direct verbal communications. Rather, interactions commenced with frequent handling of the woman's body, as the doctors conducted clinical examinations and initiated medications.

Confinement to the labour table brought both physical and psychological isolation. Like many other women, Papreen said, "I didn't see anyone in the labour room. It's only the nurse and the *ayah*. I wanted to shout and cry, but couldn't. I wanted my mother there, but couldn't tell them." The experiences of giving birth in the hospital brought to the women a feeling of a different world – a world of isolation where they sensed a smell – the smell of hospital *'huspateler gondho'*. Many women who experienced hospital birth shared their recollections of the smell of hospital. The women differentiated this unusual experience of *huspateler gondho* from the simple smell of the hospital that carried with it the odour of medicine.

The importance of women's experiential knowledge came to an end in medical encounters. In the hospital, the women were highly criticised for trying birth at home and using their own knowledge. In one labour room situation, Jorina arrived with labour pain at the THC. The nurses became very angry with them. One of them said, "After failing everything, you came to the hospital. You rustic, when will you be civilised?" The rural women possessed *moner shahosh* and *shoriler shakti* that influenced them to recognise the language of their body in childbirth experiences. They felt that these *moner shahosh* and *shoriler shakti* were no longer required in hospital birth where doctors' knowledge, technological devices and pharmaceutical measures were at hand. As Marsheeda said,

> In the hospital, you don't need *moner shahosh* or *shoriler shakti*. *Daktarnis* (female doctors) are there. They give you saline[7] to increase your *shoriler shakti*. They give you an injection to increase your pain. These saline and injections bring the baby out.

Despite their ability to understand their bodily experiences they seemed to lose it in hospital birth.

Many women who were delivered in the hospital did not understand the movement and descent of the foetus during their birthing experiences in hospital. A woman said,

> I didn't feel how the baby was born. Doctors did everything. They understand everything. They know how to deliver the baby. They know what medicine is needed. They know how to cut your stomach to bring the baby out. They have all kinds of knowledge. They gain knowledge from the book.

For their complete dependence on doctor's knowledge, women lost their intuitive power to understand bodily mechanisms during childbirth.

The nurses in the THC often incorporated the local knowledge of birth practices. A significant observation in a birth event in the THC was of a birthing woman's mother who tied an herbal root around her daughter's thigh on approval from a nurse. This family came from a better-off economic class and decided earlier to have birth in the THC. But, when the mother thought the progress of labour was delayed, she sent someone to collect herbal roots in order to hasten the labour process. At the same time, she was hesitant to tie the roots in case the nurses got annoyed. The nurse said, "It does not hamper our conducting labour. Why should we discourage it?" Correspondingly, giving sanctified water and reciting Koranic verses were also common in the THC.

Communication with Biomedical Professionals

Women's hearts sank when they encountered caregivers in hospitals and found difficulties in understanding the language spoken by these people. The language the doctors used in the hospital was urbanised and bookish, very different from the local dialects used by rural women. Shahera shared her experience,

> The doctor was telling me, '*chap dao, chap dao* (push, push)'. I thought she was asking me about the sources of drinking water. I told her that I drink water from *chap kol* (tube well). Then, she asked an *ayah* to explain this to me.

The blank faces of the women revealed that they did not understand what the doctors said about them with other doctors and nurses. One intern doctor said,

> I feel bad. I want to make patients understand, but they don't. Once I asked a patient to get a test tube, but she was not able to follow me. Later, I asked to bring a *shui* (needle) and *nol* (syringe). She brought a test tube. I get frustrated over communicating with them and lose my temper.

The doctors became annoyed when the women failed to understand their instructions, and the need for further explanations led them behave rudely with the women.

The communication of biomedical professionals with their patients was predicated on muteness among the latter. When women were keen to express their subjective experiences of physical problems, their voices were muted either by being ignored by non-response, or being abused with a harsh response, or communicating with non-understandable languages.

Patient: *Apa*, my back is hurting. I can't move my legs.
Doctor : No response, but checked foetal heart sound.
Patient: *Apa*, I am having so much pain. I can't bear it anymore.
Doctor: Didn't you remember that when you slept with your man?
Patient: *Apa*, please remove the *nol* (catheter) from my *peshaber rasta* (urinary passage)?
Doctor: You have urinary retention (In English). The catheter can't be removed.

I have observed in hospitals how women's voice in expressing their embodied knowledge was muted in their own childbirth experiences. A woman was admitted with prolonged labour pain. The doctor examined her and diagnosed intrauterine death with face presentation. On the other hand, the woman repeatedly said, "My baby is moving." The doctor said, "It's not moving." Her eyes became tearful. The intern doctors came enthusiastically in groups to see a case of face presentation. They all examined her. She seemed to be shouting with her blank stare, "My baby is moving." The *ayah* standing beside her quietly said, "Keep your patience, sister. Call the God." The baby was delivered with forceps and left on the floor in a steel tray. Suddenly, someone discovered that the baby was moving. The doctor screamed, "The baby is moving. Bring it here." She started to resuscitate the baby and later, declared it as dead. The woman was looking at the scene quietly. Like that woman, I also became a silent observer watching the scene quietly. Perhaps the baby would not have survived. But, why didn't the doctor listen to the patient from the beginning?

Doctors seemed unable to listen to patients' voices unless their problems became visibly expressed. Khaleda was diagnosed with postpartum haemorrhage. All the doctors came and examined her by removing her vaginal pack to observe the bleeding. Khaleda felt pain on each vaginal examination, "Please don't hurt me. I don't have much bleeding." Khaleda was experiencing different problem. She was developing swelling around her neck and face and feeling a choking sensation. She said, "This bleeding is normal. I am having chest compression, but no one is taking care of it." Not a single doctor listened to her problem. She attracted the doctor's attention when her condition became critical. All the doctors examining Khaleda judged her condition with the singular thinking of postpartum haemorrhage. They ignored her chest compression, as they were not ready to accept her other immediate problem until it was visibly noticeable.

The behaviour of the doctors and nurses dumbfounded the rural women. In the labour room, the birthing women were abused both verbally and physically. One birthing woman was left unattended on the labour table. Suddenly, her perineal area was bulging and the baby's head was seen. The woman started to hold her legs together to prevent the baby coming out. A doctor rushed to her scolding, "*Magi* (a prostitute), how dare you? Open up your legs." She spanked on the woman's thighs. The woman frighteningly spread open her legs and the baby came by itself. In another instance, a birthing woman was screaming due to her intolerable pain. The attending doctor spanked on her leg and shouted, "If you scream one more time, I will hit you again." The doctors were usually not aware of their own behaviour. Their offensive and crude conduct happened unknowingly and was followed by the other doctors and nurses.

One morning I sat in the antenatal ward. The doors and windows were all open. An intern doctor had begun to check all the patients. She tried to listen to the foetal heart sounds of the patients after exposing their abdomens. After examining each patient, she moved to the next. She did not bother about maintaining the privacy of the patient or making the patient feeling reassured. As one patient was not found on the bed, she became irritated, "Whenever I come, she is not in the bed." She went to the next patient and found a dirty tin bowl near her foot. She shouted, "Remove this bowl. Why did you keep it near my foot? I'll kick this bowl out." She communicated with each patient by using the word *'tumi'* (you). A patient's attendant tried to ask her something. She became annoyed, "Why did you come here? Wherever I go, this woman follows me. What a nuisance? Leave this place. I can't talk to you now?" She got irritated with each patient. The patients looked frightened and did not dare to ask any questions.

The rural women felt humiliated, insulted and sad when the doctors behaved rudely with them. Rownak's words conveyed the message,

Apa, I have shared many things about the hospital, but I didn't tell you one thing that still bothers me a lot. I will never forget the words the doctor said about the sexual relationship with my husband I didn't raise my voice, just kept quiet and wanted to come back home. I will never go back to the hospital. She has insulted my personal life.

The women did not dare to place questions before doctors and nurses in fear of getting humiliated. Romila said, "They get irritated if we ask questions and start to scold us. I feel scared to talk with them." Shaheena, a schoolteacher from *Apurbabari* shared her experiences about neglectful attitudes of the doctors and nurses towards poor patients,

Poor people suffer a lot. I observed it when I was hospitalised for my childbirth. These people do not have money and cannot buy everything on time. They are not used to live in a place like hospital. They do not understand the language. Doctors and nurses do not talk nicely with them. Knowing the situation of your profession, you have chosen to be a doctor and nurse. I teach poor students in the Primary school. I know their family status. I can't lose my temper if they can't prepare their studies, and wear dirty ragged clothes. Doctors and nurses should understand the situation of patients and develop caring attitudes. Their rude behaviour makes poor patients very sad and insulted. Most patients get partially well listening to their kind words. They don't expect much.

In fear of humiliation, information was kept hidden and instructions not followed. I observed in the Medical College Hospital that the patients did not take medicine regularly, but when the doctors and nurses enquired about it, they simply denied it. In postnatal wards many babies were fed with infant formula, but this information was also hidden from the doctors. Moreover, after having caesarean sections some women took rice and curries when they were prescribed liquid or semi-solid diet. Poor communications resulted in concealing of information and violating of instructions.

Lack of communications between caregivers and patients sometimes led to fatal consequences. An eighteen-year old girl was admitted with obstructed labour. She had a caesarean section but the baby was dead. She developed infections in her genital tract and abdomen leading to cessation of bowel movement and subsequently to lung infections and death.[8] The mother was highly criticised for giving food to the girl and blamed for causing her daughter's death. She sadly elaborated the story,

> On the third day, my daughter was given a diet of milk and sugar from the hospital. They said that it was patient's diet. Her mouth was dry. I gave her little milk and sugar to eliminate the dryness. But, on the following day, her stomach became distended. The doctor aspirated fluid from there. On the next day, worms started to come out of her mouth and choked her to death. My daughter is dead now. Why didn't they tell me not to give anything by mouth? I was scared to ask questions.

With these bitter experiences, the rural women went back home. Their stories created fright among other village women and made them disinclined to seek hospital obstetric care.

Instruments Sterilised or Washed or None?

Despite the arrangements for sterilising instruments, most of the time non-sterilised instruments, gloves and urinary catheters were used during delivery in the labour room of the hospital. Every now and then, the same non-sterilised instruments were used on different patients. The nurses imitated the doctors. I observed three patients lying on the labour tables. One set of episiotomy instruments left on the trolley was blood stained. A doctor was stitching the episiotomy incision of a patient. Suddenly, another birthing woman started to push. The doctor rushed to the patient. She asked for scissors. The special *ayahs* looked at each other. The doctor lifted the used scissors from the trolley to cut the perineal area of the patient. These were not uncommon practices observed in hospitals.

Gloves were simply washed in tap water and dried in fanned air. These gloves were regularly used while examining patients or delivering the baby. The urinary catheters were washed only in water and sometimes sterilised by immersing in antiseptic solutions. Women were catheterised with these urinary catheters. In both the Medical College Hospital and THC I observed similar practices. I saw the same needle used for two different patients. Two patients gave birth in the labour room one after the other. When a new patient was brought into the labour room, the nurse removed the intravenous saline from the first patient and inserted the same needle into the new patient.

Coconut oil was commonly used as a lubricant in the THC. The doctors, nurses and *ayahs* admitted that coconut oil was used in many different THCs instead of antiseptic solutions. While I questioned a doctor about the use of coconut oil and the chance of infections, she laughed, "*Apa*, everyone uses coconut oil in the THC." In response to my question, a nurse in the THC said, "Go and see the similar practices in the Medical College Hospital and District Hospital. Doctors do the same." However, I did not observe such practices in this Medical College Hospital.

Maintaining Privacy in Childbirth

Women's privacy was incessantly violated in an uncaring hospital atmosphere. I observed in the THC and the Medical College Hospital how medical rituals infringed woman's privacy during childbirth. Rebecca was laid down on the labour table. Her hands were strapped down because intravenous saline was being administered. Her legs remained apart, her feet were positioned by putting the steel bars of the stirrups in between her big toe and the adjacent toe, and the *saree* was folded onto her stomach exposing the whole genitalia. An intern female doctor was stitching her perineum. A senior male doctor was teaching a group of medical students. They all looked at the process of perineal stitching. Rebecca covered her face with an end of her *saree*. She appeared disgraced, numb, and motionless. In another incident,

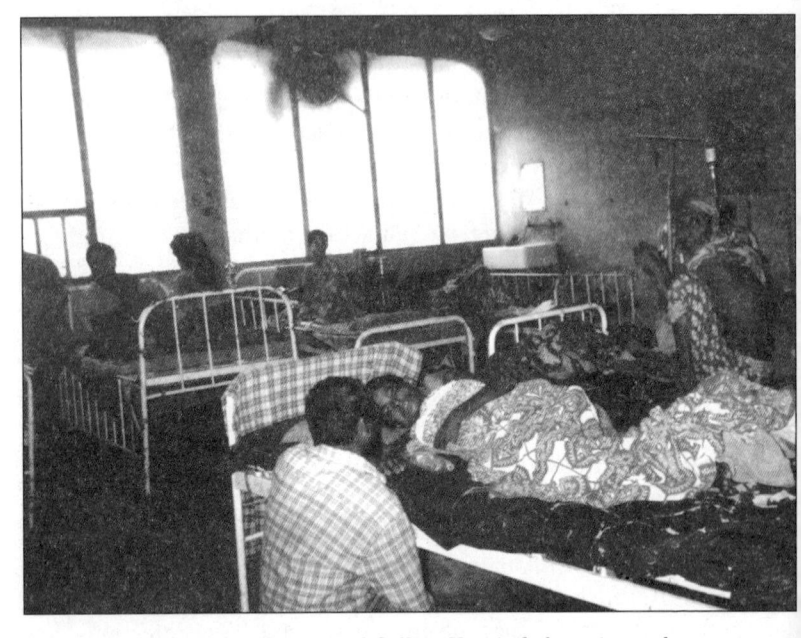

Photo 14: The Medical College Hospital obstetric ward

Samira had severe bleeding after her delivery. Doctors both male and female came into the labour room and checked her bleeding by lifting her petticoat and removing the sanitary pad. They all left her exposed without putting the pad back. Her mother standing nearby replaced the pad again and again. Samira was disgraced and upset not only for being exposed but also by being touched by male doctors. Her mother said, "Male doctors are touching her body. Who will come to the hospital again?"

Unlike other wards, the movement of men, except for male doctors, was restricted in the labour room. If a patient's male attendants tried to enter, they were immediately driven out and insulted, particularly by special *ayahs*. Yet, I observed a situation when two male plumbers entered into the labour room to fix the water tap in the basin. Two women were lying on the labour table half-naked. There was no screen or partition to keep the patients out of sight. The plumbers spent more than twenty minutes in fixing the tap. No one covered those two birthing women. A special *ayah* who regularly attended birth in the hospital said, "I won't come to the hospital for my own childbirth.

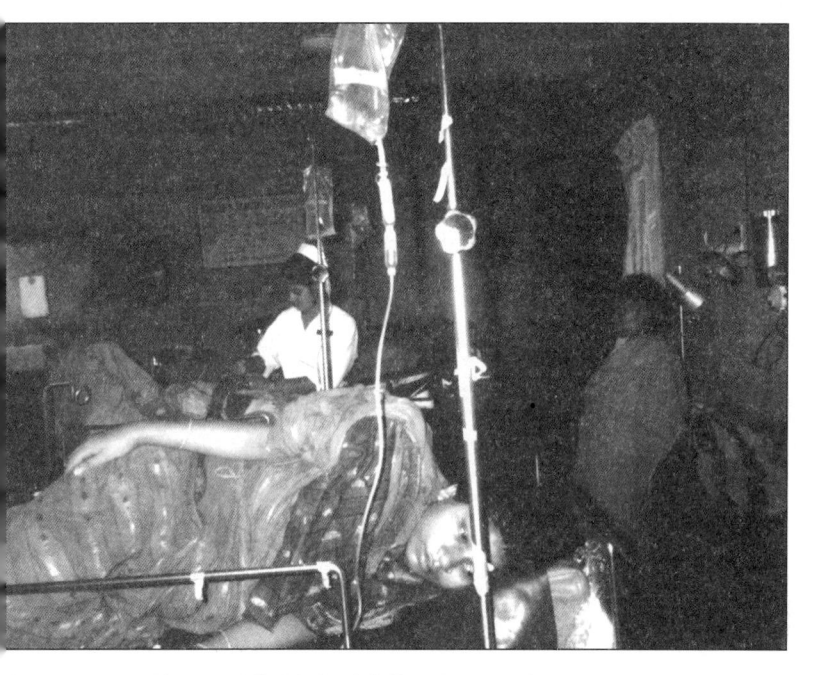

Photo 15: The Medical College Hospital labour room

There is no privacy. If someone has any sense of dignity, they won't come to the hospital for child delivery."

Rural women felt degraded and intimidated for having their private parts exposed. These issues were constantly referred to in the village, among women, as reasons for not seeking hospital care, even in emergency situations. Typically they considered it a matter of extreme *sharam*. In sum, the inappropriate behaviour of doctors and nurses created an insensitive atmosphere in the labour room that did not account for the privacy of the patients during their very intimate experiences of childbirth.

Facing Birth and Death Together

As any other hospitals, these study hospitals not only treated disease and made patients well but they also dealt with death. A very common concern among the rural women was facing the scene of death in the hospital. In the labour room, the beds were all placed side by side. Once I observed that a woman having live birth watched another woman giving stillbirth on the adjacent bed. No one attended the birth of the stillborn baby. The sight of giving stillbirth was heartbreaking and dreadful. This woman was left on the labour table at the corner of the room where the dead baby was hanging from her womb. This scene made the other woman waiting for giving live-birth emotionally uncomfortable. She covered her face with the end of a *saree*. I also observed the death of a patient in the labour room with other birthing women lying down on the adjacent beds. Apart from this, the emotional outbreaks of relatives occasioned by the death frightened other patients. Not surprisingly, this organisation of childbirth in the hospital also contributed to the reluctance of rural women to seek hospital care.

Cheating in the Hospital

Many incidents occurring in the hospital gave rise to fear. Warnings were written all over the places: "Be careful of cheats", "Do not give your medicine to any white-gowned person. Give your medicine to your nurses only", "Keep your money and ornaments carefully" and so on. Selina, a nurse from the THC, explained how an intern doctor stole medicine when her son was admitted into this hospital,

> This injection was very expensive. We bought three injections and gave to the intern doctor. On the first day, my son was given an injection and that's it. I complained to a senior doctor. After that, the intern doctor was no longer seen in that ward.

I met one patient's attendant who narrated a story where one white-gowned man tricked them,

> We thought he was a doctor. He wore a white apron and carried a stethoscope around his neck. He asked for medicine. I gave it to him. After that he never showed up. It costs us more than Tk. 300.

It was understood that a well-organised group was working in the hospital to cheat on poor, illiterate patients. When the patients came to know about cheating, they became worried about the possibilities of further cheating. These circumstances, encountered in the hospital, made them cautious about hospital environment and created resentment to seek hospital obstetric care.

Rejoicing Birth in the Hospital

In hospital, when women and babies were revived from the hazards of pregnancy-related complications, rural women, in particular, were genuinely appreciative of the success of modern hospital obstetrics. The experience of their revival made them ignore the behaviour of doctors and nurses. I met Mameena, a member of an NGO involved in the Safe Motherhood Initiatives in *Apurbabari* village. Her first, childbirth experience at home, and the last, in the hospital led her to have positive impressions about hospital birth. Mameena described in these words,

> When my first child son was born, I had difficulties. It was a breech delivery. My son was born alive, but I had developed problems in birth canal. It became swollen. It was so painful that I couldn't put any warm compression on it. Subsequently, I discovered that it came down when I lifted heavy loads or did something hastily or sat without a support at the bottom. After six years, when I got pregnant with my second child, I was physically worn out. I didn't have any physical strength to participate in labour. The experience of first childbirth and my physical weakness made me decide to seek hospital care. My husband didn't want me to go to the hospital. He believed that doctors killed his father in the hospital, as they were not able to collect money to buy medicine for him. I had to convince him that I wouldn't have any problem, as I had saved Tk. 500 by working in BRAC. In the hospital, I didn't have any problem. They put me on the bed and gave saline and injections. When I had severe pain, they came and delivered the baby by cutting my anal area.

Mameena's statement clearly conveys the message that childbirth is safely done in the hospital with reduced physiological difficulties of birthing women. Mameena's views were influenced by the discourses on seeking hospital care in birth complications. The story of her father's-in-law death and the family's disagreement could not change her frame of mind about hospital experiences. However, such positive hospital experiences are not yet part of the discourse of rural women about hospital delivery.

Experiences of Attendants: Tending Patients

From my observations it was evident that in the hospital, the female attendants nursed female patients and the male attendants carried out supportive tasks. The female attendants were mother, mother-in-law, sister, sister-in-law, daughter and female relatives and neighbours. In occasional cases, the husband and father also attended a female patient. Feeding, giving oral medications, bathing, changing and washing clothes, changing urine bags, giving bedpans and keeping eyes on blood transfusion and saline infusion were all their tasks. The male attendants included husband, father, father-in-law, brother, brother-in-law and other kinfolk. They accompanied the patients to execute various tasks, such as, buying medicine, collecting money, doing investigations, bringing blood, and getting food.

The female attendants constantly stood up on their legs to execute the tasks that were likely to be done by nurses and *ayahs*. Despite their toil, the attendants were criticised over and over again by the nurses, doctors and *ayahs*. One attendant said, "They get so annoyed with everyone. I feel scared as I don't know what mistakes I have made." In one event, a senior doctor from the Faculty of Medicine came to see a patient in an Obstetric ward. A twelve-year old girl looking after her mother stood nearby. As the doctor could not find any duty doctor, he looked into the patient's file and left the room without writing any prescription. Soon after, the two intern doctors came and started to scold the little girl for not informing them. She seemed puzzled and was unable to comprehend her mistake.

In another incident, a patient was catheterised to relieve urinary retention. The bag was full with urine. She wanted to have her catheter removed and expressed her desire to go to the toilet. Her attendant requested for my help. I suggested her to call for a nurse. The attendant said, "The nurses will not come." On my advice she went to get a doctor. She pleaded with two doctors who happened to be in the ward, "*Apa*, please come and see the patient. The bag is now full with urine. Her bladder will soon explode. Please remove the catheter." Both the doctors felt insulted, became infuriated and abused her verbally. One doctor said, "Take off the bag, empty it and then connect after a while." The other doctor made a face and imitated her intonation, "The bladder will be exploding! Didn't you get any other place to show your good acting? Bladder will be exploding, *apa*." They left without providing any assistance to the patient. The attendant looked at me perplexedly. Then, a special *ayah* came forward to help her out. Undoubtedly, she was paid.

I saw hundreds of men waiting anxiously outside the female wards either seated or stood up on the long veranda or corridor. The male attendants were seen running everywhere to execute tasks in support of the woman patients. As most rural men did not have formal education, they could not follow all the instructions. Even if some were able to read, the hospital was so big and the rooms were so scattered that assistance was required. A male attendant asked a doctor, "*Apa*, how do I collect the blood?" She described it as if the man knew the place well. The male attendants tried to avoid the assistance of *ayahs* and security guards because the latter always asked money for their service. In order to accomplish a task in the hospital, several signatures were required. The male attendants ran hither and thither with the patient's file and got harassed everywhere. On occasion, the task was not done, even after running for the whole day. As the attendants took the patient's file, the duty doctors also criticised them because they failed to refresh daily orders.

On the other hand, in the THC, nurses' behaviour with the patient's attendants was not as hierarchical as in the Medical College Hospital. The nurses had previous acquaintance with many attendants. The patients and their families, whom I met in the THC, were accompanied by individuals who already knew the hospital staff. Moreover, in this Health Complex, the Residential Medical Officer (RMO) and many nurses came from the adjacent areas and were known in the locality. Although, the attendants and nurses disputed over when medicines were bought and patients were released, rude communications were not usually observed. The villagers observed the difference between the tertiary hospital and THC. Romila's husband told, "The way the doctors behaved with us in the Medical College Hospital, if they would have done this in the THC, they faced problems."

Must We Pay the Costs?

Rural women and their families arrived at the hospital with the worry of impending hospital expenses. They had little clue about the actual expenses. When they faced it, real expenses usually exceeded their anticipated budget. In the THC, I observed that referring patients with pregnancy complications to the closest Medical College Hospital was difficult for the nurses and doctors. A woman was admitted with very high blood pressure, which was generally not treated at the THC. The nurses failed to convince the woman to seek care from the Medical College Hospital. The patient started to cry holding a nurse's hand, "Please don't send me to the big hospital. We can't afford the costs. My husband has to sell the house if we spend so much money. If I die, I will die here." Some expenses were involved in receiving treatment at the THC, but it was much lower than the costs incurred in the Medical College Hospital. Shaheron said with reference to seeking care from this hospital, "One needs more money for buying medicine, buying food and travelling. You need more people to accompany you and that involves more expense." Fear of bearing the costs of huge hospital expenditures made villagers hesitant to seek sophisticated obstetric care.

As soon as the patients arrived at the Medical College Hospital, the doctors became nervous when the patient's situation seemed serious. After examining the patient, they gave a list of medicine. At times, the doctors failed to consider the economic situation of the patient. Immediate need to buy medicine put the poor villagers under tremendous pressure to secure money by hook or by crook. In my observation, they arrived at the hospital with some cash, but the amount of money required for hospital treatment was beyond their imagination. At the same time, due to their unfamiliarity with the hospital and the surroundings, they did not know where to buy medicines. The patient's attendants were seen running nervously from here to there on their arrival. On the other hand, the doctors became impatient when they failed to buy medicines immediately. Delays in treatment made them more nervous and rude to the patient.

Even with the availability of equivalent medicine in the hospital, the intern and junior doctors prescribed medicines of different trade names that cost the poor patient a small fortune. In the hospital, one patient's husband showed me the drug list. I understood that some drugs were available in the hospital and checked with the nurse-in-charge. She said,

> We can't do anything today because I have already sent the requisition to hospital drugstore. From tomorrow, she will get medicine. The intern doctors always do the same mistake. They prescribe medicine in different trade name, but these medicines are also available in the hospital. If we send the requisition form with these trade names of medicine, the drugstore will not dispense it because the name written on the form is different.

In another event, I observed that an intern doctor hurriedly gave a drug list to a patient who was due to have Dilation and Curettage (D&C) under general anaesthesia in the same day. The nurse-in-charge was not aware of the operation, as a preoperative order was not written in the patient's file in the previous night. On my inquiry, the doctor said, "Yesterday I told the patient that she would have operation today. But, I did not write the preoperative order. I just gave them the medicine list." The patient was taken to the operating theatre. The attendant went to the drugstore to buy medicines from the list, which was just handed in. Despite the fact that some medicines were available in the hospital, the patient's attendant was asked to buy the similar medicines. The nurse said, "If the doctor had written the preoperative order last evening, the patient would have received some medicine from the hospital." Simple mistakes of the doctors contributed to the financial burden on the patient's family.

The intern and junior doctors were not always aware of trade names of all medicines, their costs and the availability in the hospital. Beside, influenced by the pharmaceutical representatives, they prescribed medicine from their companies, which were also available in the hospital drugstore in different name. At the same time, they also prescribed newly marketed, costly medicine. The pharmaceutical representatives were always seen to follow the intern doctors in the wards, duty rooms and corridors. During my thirty minutes stay in a doctor's duty room, I met five pharmaceutical representatives. All of them began to discuss the importance of a particular drug, and then, gave a gift, such as, pen, notebook and so on to each doctor. Some of them gave medicine as well. The representatives also checked their medicine list, which they previously hang on the wall of the intern doctor's room. In the wards, I observed them checking patient's medicine orders and accessing hospital registers without seeking permission from the nurses. The nurses tried to stop them, but they did not pay heed.

Getting hardly any medication from the hospital gave rise to suspicions among the patients. They suspected that doctors intentionally withheld medicine or stole medicine from their given portions. I discovered that in some cases, hospital staff or their relatives received hospital medication whereas the poor did not. It made an unpleasant impression in their mind. Besides, all over the hospital, a rumour circulated from mouth to mouth that some doctors stole medicine. The doctors acknowledged this, "Sometimes all medicines are not needed for treating patients. We save it for the poor." I remember, during my internship in the hospital, we used to save medicine from the well-off patients and the pharmaceutical companies for the donation box. In recent times, many doctors used the medicine given by pharmaceuticals as a free sample for their personal reasons. This exacerbated the suspicion of hospital doctors stealing medicine. On the other hand, doctors also started to believe that the poor villagers tried to trick them by showing their inability to buy medicine. Patients and their families accepted it as a fact that doctors would kill the patients if they failed to bring money and buy medicine. This created an environment of distrust between the patients and the doctors.

I heard everywhere that drugs were stolen from the hospital. Even though, the dispensing of drugs was restricted, theft occurred incessantly before, during and after dispensing. One doctor noted,

> The problem starts from the very beginning when the government calls for a tender from the agent. Three to four agents usually get the contract to supply drugs to the hospital and sell drugs at very high prices. No one says anything because high officials are involved in it.

In the course of discussion, another doctor said,

> The serious crime happens in the central drug store. Most drugs get stolen before their arrival in the hospital. Drugs are also stolen in hospital drug store and in dispensing. The ward boys who bring the drugs from the store also steal some. Hospital drugs are seen available in the market.

When nurses tried to identify the thief, hospital blankets were noted to have disappeared from wards. As nurses had to bear the expenses of the lost hospital goods, they accepted the reality and maintained silence. The dispensing of intravenous saline also became very restrictive. It was only dispensed after empty saline bags were returned to the hospital drugstore. As the bags were stamped with a special trademark, these could not be sold to the local drugstores but were available in the local, private clinics. Drugs were also stolen from the patients, as I witnessed in the ward when a fake doctor wearing a white-coat took drugs from a patient and disappeared. Even with all the written and verbal notices of handing in medicine only to ward nurses, poor, rural patients and their attendants always faced these situations. Doctors stealing drugs was a common tale in the hospital. The nurses muttered the names of many doctors thought to be involved in medicine stealing. I had to remain aloof because it was not my role to work as a crime investigator. Yet, my interest in this, for the purpose of the study, is that it served as yet another deterrent for the poor villagers to seek hospital care.

The urgent need for blood was a common picture in the obstetric unit. Intern doctors along with the patient's attendants started running to get blood from the hospital blood bank. However, blood was always scarce in the blood bank even with the involvement of *Shandhani*[9]. Blood bank charged each patient Tk. 200 for one bag of blood. Despite immediate payment, collecting blood on time was difficult. As a result, the patient's condition deteriorated and emergency surgery delayed. One senior doctor said, "Blood is an opportunity for the criminal. They hide blood in order to sell at high price. At night, they won't receive telephone calls and keep the door closed. In emergency, they sometimes ask for Tk. 1,000."

Despite the availability of facilities for laboratory investigations in the hospital, patients were sent to the private laboratories. Many private laboratories were located near the hospital. The pathologists and technicians working in these laboratories were all hospital employees. The patients were told, "The reagents required for investigations are not available in the hospital." As one doctor said, "It is a big profit making business. These labs earn so much money that even if their doctors get transferred elsewhere they cancel it by bribing the officials." These business ventures compelled patients to do investigations in private laboratories.

The supply of meals was inadequate in comparison to the number of patients in the Medical College Hospital. These deprived many poor patients of receiving food. But, they were afraid to challenge the criteria for receiving hospital meals. The nurses tried to distribute meals to patients by judging their economic status and the geographic distance of their residence. However, they were not always successful. One nurse commented,

> I cry when I see poor patients sitting with their plates and waiting for meals. Food is given to many patients who are related to hospital staff. When the issue was put before the Deputy Director of the hospital, he said that they were as poor as others. Yes, they are also poor, but do not live far. We can't make everything possible in spite of our willingness.

As Romila said, "I was getting bread and milk. One day I got only milk, but the other day I did not. I was not sure what my meal was." Poor patients could not even ask for fear of being insulted. She said, "If you ask, they scold you." On the other hand, the hospital dietician explained to me why the quantity of meals was insufficient. He said,

> Previously, whatever expenditures incurred in providing diet was met from the budget. The yearly budget allocates Tk. 7,200,000 for meal, but the hospital spent additional Tk. 8,000,000. The contractors were not paid and refused to supply further meals to the hospital. Then, it was decided that no more additional meals would be prepared.

The budgetary constraints deprived poor patients of receiving hospital meals.

In the hospital, I constantly heard that food was stolen and its taste was bland. Those serving meals, who happened to be *ayahs* and ward boys, were blamed for stealing and replacing meals. One doctor told me, "One can't finish the story of hospitals. Have you tasted hospital meals? Is it edible for human beings?" For my own erudition, I went to visit the kitchen. I was fascinated by what I observed there. The kitchen was absolutely clean, the cooks were neatly dressed and the flavour and texture of the food made my mouth salivate. I was even more fascinated when I spoke with the dietician, who clearly described the cooking methods and nutritional values of meals. I looked at my research assistant and came out stupefied. The meals that were served to patients seemed different. I was puzzled by the puzzle of hospital meals.

Poor patients were forced to pay for medicine, laboratory investigations, blood transfusion and foods causing huge financial burden. They had to pay money to the *ayahs*, trolley pullers and gatekeepers at different points for the simplest tasks. On refusal of payment, the patients and their families were misguided and the staff became uncooperative. In the THC, the nurses were also paid for assisting in child delivery. One doctor admitted that he used to charge patients for the delivery while working at another THC, but in this THC he did not. He said, "Patients are extremely poor in this area. I don't want to take share from the small amount of money they pay to nurses." However, he told me about his private practice in the THC outdoor during the office hour. In the context, he said, "Once a Minister came to visit our hospital. A group of people complains about the doctor's private practice. He openly criticised all of us. On his departure, he secretly told us, you continue your work. We laughed." The result was that poor patients bore all the costs to avoid troubles and to receive good treatment.

I tried to estimate total expenditures on normal birth and caesarean section from patients and their attendants' viewpoints. The estimated total costs for normal childbirth was about Tk. 800 at the THC and Tk. 1,600 at the Medical College Hospital whereas for caesarean section it was about Tk. 15,000. A study done in Dhaka city demonstrated that the total costs for normal childbirth at the hospital was Tk. 1,275 (US$31.9), and for caesarean sections Tk. 4,703 (US$ 117.5) (Nahar & Costello, 1998).

Collecting money from different sources made life difficult for the poor villagers, who usually did not have specific assets or savings. No one wanted to give a loan to these poor people. They borrowed money from the moneylenders at very high interest rates.[10] They also raised money by selling cows, goats, land and even the tin-roof of their huts. Romila's husband had saved some money to buy land for their house. All his savings were spent in the hospital for treating Romila's pregnancy complications. He also borrowed money from moneylenders. His eyes were full of tears, "Allah! Tell me how do I pay off the money?" Shaheron sighed, "If I die, I will die at my own village. I don't want my family to sleep on the street." In the end, the poor became poorer by losing their last penny for receiving hospital treatment and trapped in the cycle of poverty and malnourishment.

Getting Discharged from the Hospital

Women with a normal vaginal delivery were released 24 hours later and those who had a caesarean section after a week in the Medical College Hospital. In the THC, rural, birthing women, along with the female relatives, insisted on leaving the hospital right after the delivery. Staying in the hospital did not fit into the frame of reference of birthing women. They believed that they were unnecessarily held in the hospital, a place, which was also frightening. In hospital, they encountered difficulties while eating, sleeping and using toilets. More importantly, they had a strong desire to cleanse their body and the baby for the purification, which were difficult to execute in the hospital.

The flight of patients from the hospital was a common event. Procedural delays forced them to run away from the hospital. In the THC, I observed patients' attendants arguing with nurses to release them. A nurse explained, "Look, we can't discharge you. Only doctors can discharge a patient. Wait till the doctor comes back. He will write your patient a prescription." Even then, the attendants insisted on discharging the patient. The nurse left the place for a while. In the meantime, the patient ran away with the attendants. In *Apurbabari*, Rownak and Hamida shared their experiences of escaping from the hospital. Rownak described how they managed to escape,

> Escaping from the hospital is another story. My husband hired a tempo and left it near the rear gate. My mother-in-law went before with the clothes. I went out with my sister-in-law to have a stroll in the corridor. Then, I saw my husband signalling us to follow him. We followed him and got into the tempo. Anyway, my husband had to pay some money to the gatekeeper.

At times, they fled from the hospital to avoid payment to nurses and *ayahs*. All the issues persuaded them to leave the hospital without notifying the authorities.

Getting a discharge certificate from intern doctors was a pitiable experience for the patient and their attendants. Leaving the hospital was not a simple matter even when the senior doctors had released the patient. I observed one event in which a doctor harassed the woman and her family because she was asked to write a discharge certificate. It was five o'clock in the afternoon. The intern doctor walked along the corridor. Rehana's husband, along with few other patient's attendants, followed her imploring, "*Apa*, please write my wife's discharge certificate." The doctor became infuriated, "Will you stop following me? How can I give this if it is not written?" I followed the doctor. She entered into the intern doctor's room where she started chatting with friends. A few of them were writing discharge certificates. One doctor said, "I have gotten into such trouble today. Since this morning, they have been after me to write discharge certificates. Don't they know we have so much work to do?" Pointing her finger to a man standing near the door, she said, "Could you leave me now? I can't write you a discharge certificate. Come back tomorrow." The patients' attendants were standing outside the room waiting for the discharge certificate. Rehana's husband cried before me,

> *Apa*, I lost everything for my wife's treatment. I don't have any money to spend a day here. These doctors treat us like dogs. Not everyone should choose to be a doctor. Doctors should understand people. *Apa*, if you want to be good doctor, you have to conquer the heart of people.

The intern doctors treated patients and their families with no respect and dignity. These humiliating experiences gave rise unwillingness among rural people to seek care from the hospital.

Patients were eventually given a discharge certificate late in the evening. The consequences of not getting a discharge certificate on time were enormous for the family. Romila's husband was standing on the veranda looking at the sky with despair. He said, "Even if they write the certificate, we can't go home. It's far from here. It takes three to four hours by bus and then we have to take a rickshaw to reach home." Romila's sister-in-law said, "*Apa*, my sister was released in the morning. We won't get any food today. We don't have extra money to buy food. Perhaps they won't give us any bed to sleep in. Where do we go?" As soon as the discharge note was written on the patient's record during senior doctors' round in the morning, all the hospital services immediately ceased. Now, the patients who were on the bed, moved to the floor and the patients who received hospital diet were not given any more food. While I discussed the issue with the doctors, a senior doctor said,

> The intern doctors should write discharge certificate between 10 am and 12 pm, but they mostly write after 2 pm. I teach classes on discharge policy, but the intern doctors do not feel the importance of discharging patients on time. They are not aware of how rural patients arrive at the hospital and how and where they return. We encourage clinical assistants and junior doctors to write discharge certificates with the intern doctors. Thus, intern doctors will be embarrassed to finish the task and their burden will also be reduced. But, none of them bothers to follow our instructions.

Nevertheless, not releasing patients on time created further sufferings of patients and their families in the Medical College Hospital.

5.5 DOCTORS IN COSMOPOLITAN OBSTETRICS

Doctors in cosmopolitan obstetrics are involved in performing varied tasks with regard to managing obstetric patients. My intention is not to assess the skills of the doctors. What I intend to do is to concentrate on their role in cosmopolitan obstetrics, as practiced in the hospitals of Bangladesh. In the course of the discussion, the role of doctors will be described in relation to patient care together with their relationship with colleagues.

Doctor's Work

Hospital practice ensured that each doctor had diverse responsibilities. Their working pattern varied with their status. For example, the Head of the unit was responsible for the overall supervision of the unit, whereas clinical assistants supervised the treatment of each patient in their unit. Intern doctors took care of the assigned patients and the newly admitted patients under the supervision of a clinical assistant.

The working hours of the Head of the units varied in accordance with their overall responsibility. They arrived at the hospital before eight o'clock in the morning. In the morning shift, they attended to patients on their round between nine and ten o'clock. Before their arrival, nearly all the attendants were driven out of the ward and the main door of the wards remained locked. The registrar, clinical assistant, junior doctors and intern doctors usually accompanied the Head of the unit. They visited the patients in groups, listened to the patient briefing from the intern doctors, examined critical patients, if required, and occasionally questioned patients or their attendants. As the surgery was held in every alternate day, the senior doctors went straight to the operating theatre without visiting patients in the morning. During the surgery day, they only visited emergency patients. Apart from this, they also took classes to teach students at the Medical College. However, most of them were not available after two to three o'clock in the afternoon. In the evening, they occupied themselves with their private practice. One senior doctor said, "I have been working in this hospital for seven years. My family lives one-hour drive from here. But, I can't manage time to meet them even in two weeks. I don't know how my time flies so quickly." Their pre-occupation with work and private practice kept them busy throughout the day.

The clinical assistants were seen either in wards, or in the operating theatre, or in the labour room, or in their own room. They gave instructions to the intern doctors about patients' diagnosis and treatment, and continually communicated with the senior doctors. Clinical assistants were assigned to be on duty for twenty-four hours in the hospital, however, I observed them arriving in the morning and leaving in the afternoon or evening. Two clinical assistants were posted in one of the Obstetric units who divided their duty hours for the evening and night shifts. In the other Obstetric unit, the clinical assistant shared her duty with the registrar, especially at night. As each unit had admission and routine surgery every alternate day, at times, it became difficult to pursue their regular activities properly. One clinical assistant said,

> I didn't understand, before, the expanse of the responsibility. We are accountable for each patient's treatment. I am tired of working day and night. Almost every day we have to attend to surgery because newly admitted patients also require caesarean section. At the same, we manage patients with scarce resources. Is it possible to provide good care?

All of them stated that working long hours in the hospital, and managing poor patients with scarce resources made them physically and mentally exhausted.

The intern doctors began their day at seven in the morning and spent nearly the whole day in the hospital in spite of shifting duty in the evening and night. Each doctor was given responsibility to work in a ward or labour room or eclampsia room, or post-operative ward. During the morning shift, they tried to perform their allocated task. Although they supposedly wrote a patient's prognosis report before and refresh treatment order after the morning round, in most cases it did not happen in time. The duty doctors usually left the ward after the round was completed and moved scattered to different places in the Obstetric unit or to the far corners of the hospital. A common complaint about them was that they did not regularly refresh medicine orders in patient's file. As a result, the nurses were not able to send the medicine requisition in time. On the other hand, intern doctors said that they could not cope with their workload in the hospital wards. In each ward, more than twice the number of patients was admitted. In reference to this, Dr. Aloka said,

> Two of us work in this postnatal ward. I get frightened in the morning observing the volume of work. We attend patients, refresh orders and write the medical history on patients' files. It takes a long hour! If it's an admission day, we are also called in to assist in emergency caesarean section and on routine surgery day, we quickly move to the operating theatre. It would be possible to finish the assigned task in time, if we had not been asked to do other tasks.

During the evening shift, the intern doctors were not usually seen in the wards. Most gathered in the doctor's duty room and the common room writing discharge certificates and chatting. They also performed their duties from there. The intern doctors who had evening duty spent the day in the hospital from seven in the morning to midnight. The night doctors were not able to return to their residence in the following morning and spent the whole morning and afternoon for hospital duty.

On one night about ten o'clock, I observed the duty doctor checking patients in a postnatal ward. At this hour, some patients were sleeping, and some resting and chatting. The clinical assistant joined the duty doctor waking the patients who had fallen asleep and briefly examining some patients. They also refreshed medicine order and wrote out the required medicine on a piece of paper. The male attendant was immediately called in and handed the medicine list. The nurse-in-charge remarked, "I don't know when they will buy the injection and when I will push it." The doctors were seen leaving the ward after completing the night round around eleven o'clock.

After finishing medical school, intern doctors began their training period with joy, but working in the Obstetric unit devastated them. Dr. Rumana, an intern doctor whom I met in the evening shift said, "I couldn't go back to my room today because the woman admitted with incomplete abortion and cardiac incompetence in our unit was really in bad condition. Our madam (head of the unit) asked me to look after her." I remembered the patient in the labour room who was admitted on the previous night with vaginal bleeding. In the morning all the doctors, including the registrar and the clinical assistant, were seen running all over the place. The Head of the unit came to visit the patient. She asked for gloves, but none was available. The nurse-in-charge brought a pair of fresh gloves. She asked the doctors about the patient's condition. No one was able to tell the history to her satisfaction. She performed a vaginal examination and looked at the patient's file. The Head became very annoyed, and looked for the intern doctor who was on duty at that time. She said, "Where is the doctor? She didn't make any input/output chart for a cardiac patient. Tell her, I am very unhappy with her performance." The intern doctor became very upset. She later told me, "I was not told to make input/output chart. In Medicine ward, I managed cardiac patient. I was not sure what to do with this patient." Even with their effort to care patients throughout the day, they remained confused about managing obstetric complications. All the staff appeared to be stressed in the atmosphere under which they worked. This situation eventually affected patient care.

In Their Own World

In hospitals, doctors were absorbed into a world in which their own interests and understandings were seen as paramount. Preoccupation with their knowledge put emphasis on conducting childbirth under medical care. The doctors accentuated the worth of institutionalising childbirth. For example, one doctor commented: "Do you know women in any civilised country having homebirth?" Accepting the modern way of conducting birth in the hospital meant to them that one was no longer ignorant and uncivilised. Their absolute trust in hospital obstetric care as risk-free was readily apparent. On the other hand, the practices of TBAs were highly criticised by most medical doctors and considered as 'high risk'. While I was talking to a male doctor in the THC, he said, "TBAs absolutely don't know anything. Sitting before the birth canal and holding the baby after it is born. Do you consider that a skill?" This male doctor's negative attitude towards indigenous knowledge was obvious in his authoritarian tone. This attitude was spreading. The educated women in *Apurbabari* village were already convinced that a medically supervised birth is progressive and risk-free. They were delivered either in the hospital or at home with the assistance of nurses. Correspondingly, a few illiterate, rural women had also begun to see hospital birth as a risk-free practice, in spite of their very low participation in cosmopolitan obstetric care. The authority of biomedical knowledge is already encroaching on indigenous birth practices regardless of the socio-economic and cultural context of rural people in Bangladesh.

The number of caesarean sections seemed to be high in this Medical College Hospital. About forty-four percent of women admitted for obstetric reasons underwent caesarean section in this hospital, whereas the population-based caesarean section rate was 2.2 percent (Khan, Khanam, Nahar, Nasrin & Rahman, 2000). When I discussed this with doctors, a customary response was, "Prolonged labour causes cerebral insufficiency. We can't take any risk nowadays." Interestingly, more than two decades ago, the caesarean section rate was very low in the same hospital. A nurse working in the hospital said, "In 1977, each week two to three caesarean sections were done, but everyday about twenty normal births took place. But it has changed now." The increasing trend of caesarean section began out of necessity, as the biomedical professionals noted. One doctor firmly said, "It has increased because it is needed." The understanding of the doctors affirmed the need for surgical interventions. Hence, questioning the issue seemed meaningless and illogical.

I was allowed to sit in a class test of the final year medical students. The test was held in a postnatal ward. Each student was assigned to a patient to elicit the diagnosis and appropriate treatment. The examiner was the Professor of the department who took a bedside, oral examination. She listened carefully to the diagnosis and treatment of each patient from the students. She asked almost everyone about the costs of treatment in consideration of hospital expenditures.

Prof: Why do you want to do all the investigations in post-partum period?

Student: But, these investigations are important for the patient.

Prof: Yes, I understand, but you have to remember hospital expenditures incurred for it. How will the government pay for this?

Within this discussion, I never heard about the consideration of patient's socio-economic status. But, in our personal conversation the Professor commented, "The young intern doctors don't understand the patient's economic situation. They are mostly the children of elite families. You will be surprised to see their room in student dorm. All are furnished with fridge and microwave." I understood that her personal sensitivity was not reflected in her teaching because the medical curriculum does not consider patients' personal accounts.

Mother Teresa in Cosmopolitan Obstetric Care

When Mother Teresa walked along the hospital corridors to attend to patients, by and large, she was unaccompanied. The internationally known Mother Teresa[11] is no longer alive; she was not a doctor; and she never worked in a Bangladeshi hospital. The woman I am referring to as Mother Teresa was an Obstetrician in the Medical College Hospital. She was named as Mother Teresa by patients and hospital staff for her contribution to the welfare of poor patients. Before her morning round, the wards were made clean, the attendants were asked to leave the ward and the main door remained locked. The duty doctors followed her inside the wards along with the nurses. In her medical encounter with a patient:

Doctor: *Ma* (mother), how are you feeling today?

Patient: No response.

I observed that the patient was a bit surprised at her kind voice. However, she did not wait for the patient's response. The intern doctors and the nurse briefed her about the patient by looking at the laboratory investigation reports and treatment chart. She looked serious giving instructions to the doctors and nurses. If patients were unable to afford the expenditures, she tried to manage it. She could not spend more than two to three minutes with each patient, as she had to see hundreds each day. She tried to be polite and sympathetic to each patient. She wanted to be a Mother Teresa, but the reality of hospital procedures and the demands on her time did not allow her. After the patient round, the duty doctors in her ward started to refresh the treatment schedule and did their routine work, such as, writing medicine lists for the patients on a piece of paper, initiating blood transfusions, changing dressings, writing discharge certificates and so on. The doctors working in her unit tried to be dutiful. Yet, most doctors talked behind her back, "Madam spoils her patients."

Voice of Intern Doctors

The majority of the doctors came from well-off urban families. They were able to get admission to the Medical College because of their excellent academic performance. In student life they all worked very hard to obtain their degrees and dreamt of becoming a famous doctor. Dr. Neela said, "I thought it would be so nice, once I got my degree, to work in the hospital. But, working in the hospital is so different." As interns, when they faced the realities in the hospital with the treatment of patients, their dream changed. As Dr. Lily described,

> In the hospital, the drug supply is inadequate or not available. Poor people cannot buy drugs, but without drugs, we cannot treat them. Sometimes, you know, even if they have money, they don't want to spend it. They wait. When the situation of patient becomes worse, they will buy medicine. If they have money, why didn't they buy medicine earlier? For everything, either we have to collect or push the attendants to buy them.

When I first met Dr. Lucky, she was organising a drug-box maintained for the poor patients. She said, "This box is reserved for the critical patients. Our madam (Head of the unit) contributes to this from her personal reserve. She collects drugs mostly from the pharmaceutical companies." All of them stated that they encountered difficulties in treating poor patients.

The intern doctors became disappointed with their communication problems with rural patients. Dr. Naila said, "They don't understand our language and we don't understand them. How frustrating it is! Sometimes I wonder, why did I become a doctor when I can't even communicate with patients?" During our conversation, I could not resist myself from asking them why they used the word *'tumi'* (you) with each patient. She started laughing, "We feel very close. This makes us to say *tumi* to them." In Bangladesh, this form of address with the seniors (except intimately related) or the strangers indicates derogatory.

Silent conflicts were apparent between intern doctors and their immediate supervising doctors. Starting their first job with excessive workloads of obstetric patients made the new intern doctors both physically and mentally exhausted. They began to feel that their bosses intentionally pressurised them. At the same time, the supervising doctors felt that the new intern doctors tended to avoid their assigned duties. As a novice, the intern doctors were not capable of performing all the assigned tasks, but, they tried not to seek assistance of senior doctors to avoid their criticisms. Concurrently, seeking help from nurses was also felt to be unbecoming of a doctor. In the labour room, I observed a clinical assistant criticising an intern doctor for seeking a nurse's assistance, "What kind of doctor are you that you don't know how to push intravenous saline?"

In the hospital, everything seemed cumbersome to intern doctors. One said, "I think, I made a mistake by doing major in Obstetrics and Gynaecology. I will probably change it in future." Another asked me whether I would be able to give her a job in the organisation where I worked. She found my job more relaxing – only sitting in the hospital and talking to people. In the beginning of their career, lack of hospital supplies, workloads, suspicion and criticisms all worked together to create frustrations and reduce commitment among intern doctors. This eventually led to poor patient care.

Doctor's Resentment

Many doctors were frustrated for not being promoted to a higher position. Being engaged in rural or semi-urban health centres, they were not able to pursue their higher degrees. As one doctor said, "What did I get in spite of working in health centres for more than twenty years? If I had not worked here and had sat in the Postgraduate Institute Library, I would have been promoted to a higher level." This was a sad part of the story of doctors who spent years working in rural areas but were not upgraded. Promotion is usually based on the level of higher educational qualifications, not on the basis of commitment to work. Work experience does count, but by the time they receive promotion, doctors without higher degrees reach retiring age. As a consequence, the job dissatisfaction created professional jealousy and brought resentment to work that impeded the improvement of service quality in the hospital.

Many doctors were seen to feel threatened on the appointment of a new doctor who might be a competitor in their private business. A senior doctor spoke about how her colleagues, who tried to ruin her reputation. She shared her experience,

> I was doing a caesarean section on a hospital staff member's wife. The baby had foetal distress. I went to manage the baby. When I came back to my patient, I saw a new face near the operating table. I had a doubt. I started to close the abdomen. Suddenly, I remembered my friend's

words about how she was humiliated by leaving a mop[12] in the patient's abdomen. I usually don't use a mop in my operation. I asked my assistants whether they had counted the mops. None of them answered to my question. I opened abdomen again. I found a mop just behind the uterus. I just told my assistants, "Did you forget how to count?" Then I closed the abdomen. When I finished with the operation I felt drained. Someone wanted to sabotage me. But, God saved me from the mishap. I have decided at once not to do any more operations in that hospital.

Rivalry between colleagues may lead to serious negative consequence of patients and eventually affected the repute of the organisation.

Individual initiatives to bring changes in hospital quality created jealousy among colleagues and impeded the process of the venture. One senior doctor's dedication to improving service quality was not appreciated by her colleagues. Her involvement in a quality improvement project of nurses was highly criticised by other doctors. She was not only condemned, but was also thwarted not to participate in any initiative where her efforts received recognition. One doctor commented, "Does she want to be a nurse?" Doctors considered interactions with nurses as demeaning due to the latter's lowly status. However, this senior doctor was successful not only in gaining respect and love of her junior colleagues and other hospital staff, but she also succeeded in developing her career. Her success made others deliberately create problems when she tried to provide better services to patients. Jealousy and rivalry among doctors resulted in poor service quality that affected obstetric care for the rural, poor patients.

5.6 NURSES ATTENDING WARDS

Patient care depends on the nurses' role in hospital wards. Nurses perform various tasks in hospitals. Their interpersonal relationships with colleagues and doctors influence the quality of patient care. In this section, I will describe nurse's work, nursing of patients and their interactions with doctors and nurses.

Nurses' Work

Patients frequently commented on, "Nurses are always occupied with work in hospital wards." The hospital nurses in white *sarees* and student nurses in white *shalwar*[13] and *kameez*[14] were seen working in the wards, labour room, and operating theatre, doing deskwork and chatting in the duty room and walking hastily along the hospital corridors. Apart from nursing of patients, they were engaged in bookkeeping pertaining to medicine, food, and bed linens. They prepared bandages, swabs and cotton balls, received phone calls and responded to attendant's queries. Some, but not all of the nurses were always found inside the ward during their duty hours. Ashapurna, a staff nurse, proudly said, "You will only find these white dressed women always working in the ward. Our white uniform makes us easily recognisable."

I note that in different obstetric wards the duty of the nurse-in-charge of each shift started with taking charge from the previous one. Specifically, she settled up accounts of medicine and linens. In the morning, in particular, they were particularly occupied with keeping records of linen, as one nurse said, "We carefully count the linen. If stolen or misplaced, we have got to pay for this." In the wards, during evening and night, the duty hours were not as busy as in the morning, but duty in the labour room and operating theatre kept them always busy.

When student nurses were placed with the staff nurses, the former nurses were seen to distribute medicine, to clip up investigation reports in patient's file, and to send routine urine and stool examination of each patient. The student nurses, therefore, attended patients in a disgruntled manner. From what I observed, it was apparent that senior nurses tried to impose all the work directly related to patient care onto junior nurses. One senior nursing supervisor said, "We have constantly asked the senior nurses to work closely with the juniors, but they do not pay attention to us. They send the student only to distribute medicine to patients. The students get bored." Moreover, some senior nurses were seen to spend hours doing their personal jobs instead of doing their duty in the hospital wards. This behaviour was transmitted to student nurses and developed neglectful attitudes to patients. Thus, when student nurses asked for a break for genuine reasons, the senior nurses felt reluctant to approve of their request. This conflicting attitude between nurses eventually affected the service quality of the hospital.

The following narrative was an example of the working relationship among nurses and between nurses and unit doctors. I was sitting in a postnatal ward in the morning. Two staff nurses were on duty with the nurse-in-charge. The nurse-in-charge along with one staff nurse did deskwork, attended patients for medications, sent medicine and diet requisitions, and talked patiently with patient's attendants. The other staff nurse spent the whole period sitting inside the duty room. Mahmuda, the nurse-in-charge was annoyed bitterly saying, "Why do we have to be asked to do our task? We all know our duties. If all of us work equally, each patient would receive quality services within these resources." While attending patients, she discovered that the medicine orders were not refreshed. She felt disturbed with doctors who had not refreshed the daily medicine orders. Mahmuda explained the situation,

> See with your own eyes, what happens when doctors do not refresh the treatment order. Now, I cannot send a fresh medicine requisition. I have to send the previous one. Nurses are not allowed to write medicine lists for patients that are not available in the hospital. But, one's treatment cannot wait. Now, I have to write their medicine lists too. Look, some patients' diets need to be changed. These are not done yet. That means, we have to continue with the old order.

Her frustrations were caused by events, which were avoidable. As she stated, "These wrongdoings were all human-made and could easily be remedied if we all become aware." She stressed on the importance of each staff's sense of responsibility that would improve service quality and patient care.

Nursing of Patients

Nurses have a significant role to play in patient's lives, but many events in the hospital revealed their attitudinal problems toward patients and their attendants. Over and over again my observation revealed neglectful and uncaring attitudes of the nurses towards patients. A post-partum eclamptic patient was recovering from her illness. She was lying on the bed with her baby. Her husband was standing close to her, when suddenly the patient fell down from the bed. She got injuries on her head and lips. Her lower lip was bleeding and the urinary catheter was disconnected from the bag. A nurse working in the ward did not come forward, but just threw a piece of cotton to the patient and told her husband, "What are you doing there? Wipe her blood." The catheter was displaced. The nurse pushed the catheter with her feet. A doctor working for a different Obstetric unit left the ward without looking back. The husband put his wife back onto the bed. The patient said, "I wanted to lift my baby."

The nurses constantly criticised the patients and their attendants when they asked for medicine or administering intravenous saline. In one instance, an old man brought blood and some injectable medicines and asked a student nurse to help the patient. The nurse rudely said, "Get a doctor." The old man said, "I can't find the doctor." The nurse retorted, "We don't transfuse blood. Leave it there. Go away and fall sleep if you don't find the doctor." The man wanted to say something, but the nurse started to shout, "Will you get out of here?" He sadly left the place taking the medicine and blood with him. The student nurse still sat on her chair.

However, stories of uncaring neglect were interspersed with tremendous acts of kindness. I met a nurse in the THC who accompanied a poor, rural woman with birth complications to the Medical College Hospital. Shubarnalata, a nurse-in-charge explained,

> Her husband abandoned this woman. Only the old father was with her. They don't know anything about the hospital. I felt bad seeing their situation. My sister was also a nurse in Medical College Hospital. I was hoping to get some assistance from her. Yet, we had problems in the hospital. The woman had a caesarean section. The father was not well off. We all had to help them.

It was not a common event. However, such sympathetic attitudes of nurses made many poor patients grateful to them.

The interactions of nurses with the patients worried senior nurses and some senior doctors. A very senior nurse said in frustration,

> The situation of nurses is similar to a *shakher korat*[15]. There's nowhere for them to go. Nursing care to the patient is based in giving medicine, food and personal care. But, the supply of medicine and food is scarce in the hospital and the shortage of staff is quite evident. Nurses deal with patients directly. Because of this shortage, they cannot provide proper patient care. So, they start to behave badly with patients and attendants when they are asked simple questions.

I came to know from the instructors of the Nursing Institution about the ongoing projects on leadership development and quality improvement, which addressed the issues of behaviour and communications of nurses. During my fieldwork, I observed them coming to the hospital and demonstrating to student nurses the ways of improving communications and patient care.

Interactions with Doctors

The relationships between nurses and doctors were very hierarchical. Even, the intern doctors attempted the top-down approach by ignoring the age and seniority of nurses. One nurse spoke about a male intern doctor's attitudes to nurses,

> The doctor told me, not to call him *bhai* (brother) but 'Sir'. I said, you are not a professor. He said, I will be one day. Can you imagine how I felt then? I saw him as a young student.

Getting orders from intern doctors also insulted and hurt them. As one nurse said,

> The intern doctors only give you orders, bring cotton, bring gloves, bring this and that. You can tell the difference between an order and a request by looking at their faces and listening to the voice. We know how to push injections, do catheterisation and many other things better than them. But they don't call us because of their superiority complex, and just cause suffering to the patient. We can work as a team. But, they like only to give order and order.

This interpersonal relationship made nurses ignore the doctors. Sometimes, during patient management, nurses simply disappeared from the scene or engaged themselves in other activities. As a result, the intern doctors tried to keep distance by managing patients on their own or took help from hospital *ayahs* instead of asking the nurses. Alarmed by the disturbing scenes of poor nursing communication, a senior doctor got involved in some projects related to improvements in nursing, but the censorial attitudes of other doctors compelled her to stop.

The student nurses suffered most. They encountered problems in their interactions with senior nurses and intern doctors. I observed in the labour room that the intern doctors never sought help from student nurses rather they asked special *ayahs* to assist them. The student nurses were also unhappy about this relationship. One student nurse said,

> We are also here to learn, but the doctors never call us. One student has to perform ten vaginal deliveries. We deliver babies at night when the doctors sleep. In THCs and in many District Hospital, doctors don't stay. Only nurses conduct deliveries there. If we can't learn now, how will we be working there?

Not only did doctors neglect the nurses, but also a tense situation existed in their relationship where tolerance for each other was extremely poor. As a consequence, the patients suffered.

5.7 SPECIAL *AYAH'S* EXPERIENCES: SILENT SUFFERINGS

In the Medical College Hospital, two types of *ayahs* existed – special *ayahs* and government ayahs. Special *ayahs* were not government employees. These women worked in hospitals out of economic necessity and earned money by tending patients doing all kinds of menial tasks. In order to work in hospital, they perform different kinds of tasks and follow orders of all hospital staff.

In the labour room, the special *ayahs* stood beside a patient giving her physical and emotional supports as well as cleansing birth substances. In the ward, they attended the patients to feed and wash them, to wash their clothes and to cleanse faeces and urine. Apart from this, these *ayahs* maintained cleanliness in Obstetric wards.

Patients coming from rural areas sought special *ayahs*' assistance, as they were not familiar with the hospital or how to nurse patients. The problems arose when *ayahs* demanded cash for each task. Most patients were as poor as the special *ayah*. Bearing hospital expenditures along with the *ayah's* demands became a torture for them. In one instance of childbirth, the special *ayahs* assisted in child delivery and cleansing birth substances, but the patient's relatives refused to pay. The *ayahs* united, hid the patient's file and forced the patient's relatives to pay them. It was not a large amount of money, but payment for each task became a relatively large amount of money for a poor patient.

To stay and work in the hospital, the special *ayahs* did all the work imposed on them by maintaining silence. They performed all the tasks of government *ayahs*. They were the ones who washed hospital floors, walls and furniture. The *ayahs* distributed medicines among patients with nurses and meals with government *ayahs*. They also carried out heat coagulation tests on urine. I observed in the hospital that they were very intimate to new intern doctors. The intern doctors accepted the assistance of the *ayahs* during child delivery. As a novice, they did not want to reveal their ignorance, especially before senior nurses, and took refuge in *ayahs*. Yet, the senior doctors highly criticised special *ayahs* referring them as *huspateler jonjal* (hospital rubbish).

The continual presence of special *ayahs* in the labour room gave rise to a situation that went against the normal hospital procedures. I heard that when doctors or nurses were not in labour room, the special *ayahs* engaged themselves in doing vaginal examinations and delivering the baby. Once they were expelled from the hospital, as one *ayah* was caught up in the labour room doing vaginal examinations. A senior doctor said,

Everything went well in their absence. They create many problems. They were seen to increase the rate of intravenous oxytocin drip to enhance the labour process. They did that in order to demand cash from the patient's relatives for conducting the delivery.

These *ayahs* were accused of doing mismanagement in labour room and wards and creating a chaotic environment in hospital.

The special *ayahs* were exploited by the supervising staff – ward boys, ward masters, and *sarders*. I came to know from *ayahs*, nurses and also a few doctors that they had to pay at all levels not only monetarily, but also sexually. The *ayahs* talked about the physical tortures inflicted by their supervisors. They sent money to their family at home and were not able to give the shares to their supervisors, which led to this physical torture. Many of them were married-off to their supervisors. One senior doctor showed her concern about the sexual exploitation of *ayahs*. She said, "At night, you will see what *ayahs* have to pay to stay in the hospital. It is not only the lower class staff, sometimes they sleep with senior staff too." Even then, the *ayahs* were thrown out of the hospital at any time if the interests of their supervisors were impeded.

5.8 COSMOPOLITAN OBSTETRICS IN VILLAGE LANDSCAPE

The field paraprofessionals and the community health workers are a new generation of practitioners providing modern obstetric care in *Apurbabari* village. The field paraprofessionals included both NGO and government employed workers. NGO paraprofessional primarily worked in this village to render antenatal and postnatal care. The government health workers, such as health assistant (HA) and family welfare visitor (FWA) only carried out immunisation of pregnant women and infants in the antenatal care centre. The community health worker known as *shasthya kormi* (SK)[16] was involved in assisting NGO-run community activities. The SKs assisted the NGO paraprofessional in organising antenatal care centres, visited postpartum women, recorded birth-weight, conducted growth monitoring[17] and maintained information in registers. Apart from these activities, they referred patients to the NGO health centre, gave medications to TB patients, and recorded information on family planning and births and deaths.

The field paraprofessionals were trained to provide antenatal and postnatal care. Basic clinical examinations and spot laboratory investigations (urine for albumin and sugar) were carried out in antenatal care centres. After the baby was born, they paid a visit to women in their house, took blood pressure and inquired about problems of the mother and the baby. If a problem was identified, they prescribed basic medicine and advised them to seek care from the NGO run health centre or the THC. In reference to maternal, health-related activities, she said (laughingly), "Our village women are still ignorant. They don't understand much and don't show any interest to attend the antenatal care centre. We try to motivate them to attend the sessions and to have the tetanus toxoid vaccine." Antenatal care was given free at the beginning of the programme, but now, rural women obtained services with a nominal fee.[18]

As this NGO gradually curtailed down their community maternity activities, the interaction of the field professional with rural women was also reduced. Few women complained, "This *apa* does not visit as much as the previous one. The other *apa* used to discuss pregnancy related issues and spend much time with us." The field paraprofessional shared the same view, "Our field activities have been reduced. The working area is much bigger now. I can't stay longer in one village. I look after 15-20 villages." Apart from her involvement in antenatal and postnatal care, she supervised the activities of the community health workers. The field paraprofessional commented about referring patients to the health centre, "It is a headache to us. To sustain our health centre, we are given the responsibility to ensure patient flow from each village." Similarly, the community health workers stated that searching patients became a major task at present. These activities reduced their involvement with maternal health-related activities.

The community health workers were supposed to work in their own village. However, the one working in this village came from an adjacent village. At the beginning of the programme in 1992, this woman started to work in two villages due to unavailability of qualified women.[19] Subsequently, when a woman from this village was trained, she was sent to the adjacent village, but the former remained at the same place. This community health worker was Momful. She also received TBA training and started to assist in deliveries among neighbours and relatives in her own village. She insisted on the increasing willingness among pregnant women to attend the antenatal care centre, "Women are now aware about pregnancy problems. They willingly come to the centre." However, I observed in this village and other villages how the health workers continually persuaded village women to attend the centre. Momful again added, "Women are very keen to take tetanus toxoid because we have observed its effect among women and children. Nowadays, we don't hear about tetanus cases or deaths in this village." This woman tried hard to perform her assigned activities in the village. In everyday life, the community health worker was seen motivating women to attend the antenatal care centre, take vaccine and seek obstetric care if problems arose.

Although Momful assisted in childbirth, she did not consider herself as efficient as other *dainis*. She described the skills of another *daini* who worked in her own village for more than 30 years. She said,

> This *daini* called Sharnarupa is experienced and also received training seven years ago. She knows how to deal with pregnancy problem. I saw this with my own eyes how confident she was. She understands which birth she can manage and which one she cannot. Once, I was not able to deliver a baby, as it seemed to get stuck. I called Sharnarupa and at the same time, decided to send this woman to the THC. Sharnarupa inserted her hand and said that she could handle the problem. She turned the baby's head slowly and within 15 minutes, the baby was born. Not all *dainis* are as efficient as Sharnarupa.

Despite her practice as a *daini* and deep reliance on Sharnarupa, she believed that hospital was the safest place for delivering baby. Momful said, "I would not let my daughters give birth at home. I took one of my daughters straight to the hospital when she developed labour pain." But, I found out that her daughter's birth was also tried first at her husband's home, which was only one kilometre away from the Medical College Hospital. She was taken to the hospital when all home trials failed including intravenous oxytocin. This community health worker practiced as a *daini* in the village and appreciated the skills of another village *daini*, but at the same time, preferred her daughters to have hospital birth. Her conflicting attitude was created because she was encountering indigenous birth practices, but was simultaneously influenced by modern obstetric practices.

5.9 SUMMARY AND CONCLUSION

In this chapter, cosmopolitan obstetrics has been explored from the various perspectives of women, doctors, nurses, attendants, special *ayahs* and other hospital staff. In addition, fieldworkers' perspectives about birth practices were highlighted. Essentially, women's accounts of their birth experiences combined with my own observations have been triangulated to produce a detailed documentation of hospital birth. Decision-making in seeking hospital care was influenced by women's experiences as well as others. In seeking hospital care, rural, poor women and their families continued to encounter problems from getting admission to their discharge. Running hither and thither, doctors' attitudes, nurses' behaviour, huge expenditures, unfamiliar environment, and the actual experience of birth produced bitter feelings about hospital care. The experience of birth was totally different from their personal experience in homebirth. Confinement to a labour table, administration of medicine, manipulation and mutilation of the birth canal, abusive communications and lack of privacy made women silent, but humiliated and disgraced. Their passive role in hospital birth made them unimportant in their own birth experience.

Lack of supplies in hospitals gave rise to worries among women and their families and pressurised them into the urgent collection of money. This sometimes led them to spend their meagre savings and forced them into debt. Even within the framework of limited supplies, stealing of drugs, foods, blood, laboratory reagents and logistic supplies were a continual act. Moreover, the pharmaceutical representatives also played a part in influencing doctors to prescribe their drugs. All the factors contribute to huge expenditures incurred in hospital treatment.

The behaviour of the intern doctors was, in part, related to their inability to treat patients because of scare resources. Their anguish and annoyance was directed at poor patients who failed to provide the supplies in time. Not only could doctors not achieve in their proper treatment of patients, but they were also criticised by their supervisors. Nurses directly involved in patient care were abusive in their approach to patients. Neglectful attitudes were revealed in their interactions with patients and their attendants. These patterns of communication were also traced to lack of hospital supplies and at the same time, revealed the antagonism between nurses and doctors and juniors and seniors. This is a portrayal of hospital situations in which rural, poor patients experience hospital birth.

In *Apurbabari* village, the field workers tried to bring changes in the existing birth practices. Their participation, particularly in antenatal care, identified pregnant women at risk, and motivated them to seek hospital care. However, they did not fit into rural women's understanding of the world. On the other hand, the community health workers themselves suffered from a dilemma of their position.

Some of rural women's perspectives about hospital birth have been substantiated in findings of neglectful and uncaring hospital practices. Although these are punctuated with enormous acts of care by some staff, the general picture is one of systemic problems from a patient's perspective. It is not my intention at this juncture to pass judgment on what I heard and observed. Rather, the purpose of this chapter has been to show how the realities and perceptions of hospital care work to deter rural women from attending hospital in case of birth complications.

Rural women's hospital birth was not only related to their isolation in own birthing experience, but all the related incidents including involvement of doctors and nurses and the current financial deficient situation of the hospital with mismanagement and corrupt practices contribute to the construction of their hospital birth experience.

In the following chapter, childbirth practices will be analysed by situating in a multidimensional framework encompassing culture, gender, socio-economic, political economy and historical perspectives.

Notes

1 In many countries, especially in the West, white is considered as a top colour, which indicates the colour of priestly vestments and symbolises refinement and purity (Wagner, 1997).

2 One prime rule of medical profession is not to criticise other doctors or medical authoritative knowledge. If doctors defy it, they are regarded as a traitor to the profession (Wagner, 1997).

3 My husband did his PhD in Carlton University, Ottawa.

4 I have used the word 'flood' not only to signify the numbers but also the torments people face in the hospital similar to the sufferings of deluge.

5 In the eclampsia room, apart from eclamptic patients, other serious patients were also admitted. Thus, the eclampsia room was turned into an intensive care unit, as it had in-built oxygen supply. As the patients' conditions were grave, the attendants were always there by the patients. Thus, instead of being quiet, this room was extremely busy and hectic.

6 Similar issues were raised by women in another research conducted in Bangladesh (Afsana & Rashid, 2000).

7 It is important to note how women feel the importance of using saline. Intravenous saline is seen as a magic medicine that instantly brings about physical energy and hence, for any physical weakness, saline is of tremendous value to people in rural Bangladesh.

8 The woman was admitted with obstructed labour with genital infections. After caesarean section, she developed peritonitis and paralytic ileus, and subsequently aspiration pneumonea and death.

9 *Shandhani* is an organisation initiated by the student doctors for donating free blood to the patients. They charged Tk. 100 for blood grouping and cross-matching.

10 If the money were not paid off in time, it would be tripled within 6 months.

11 Mother Teresa was a Noble Prize Laureate for Peace. She devoted her life to work for the poor and sick in India as a Christian missionary.

12 Mop is a piece of cloth used to wipe blood from the abdomen.

13 *Shalwar* is a kind of loose pant

14 *Kameez* is a knee-length top.

15 It is a proverb that means any object whose presence or absence is equally painful.

16 Although the SK is a community health worker, they receive a monthly salary of Tk 600 from the NGO.

17 Infants born with low birth weight are included in food supplementation programme where they are given meals each morning and weighed each month till expected weight is reached. Few village women assist SK in organising food distribution session. These women prepare meals for the infants and earn some money by selling it to the NGO.

18 The amount of fees varied with the socio-economic conditions.

19 Their expected level of education is class VIII, but lack of educated women to work as a SK compels the NGO to select less educated women.

Chapter 6

Anatomies of Birth

> Childbirth is an intimate
> and complex transaction
> whose topic is physiological
> and whose language
> is cultural.
> – *Brigitte Jordan, 1983, p.1*

Few dispute the complexities of childbirth. Childbirth is not only a biological phenomenon but also is socially marked and shaped (Jordan, 1983; Kay, 1982; Kitzinger, 1982; MacCormack, 1982; Rothman, 1982). One of the central queries of my research has been to explore why and in what ways poor, rural women in Bangladesh adhere to indigenous birth practices and resist cosmopolitan obstetric care. As a consequence, the chapters on indigenous and cosmopolitan birth practices have provided both as Martin (1990) calls it an "ethnographic gaze" (p. 70) and, an "ethnographic ear" (p.70) in which the voice pervades and situates the findings. However, this is not enough because "order" (p. 183) is implicit in everyday practice (Smith, 1987). This means that we are in a position to "look out ... from where our respondents are and place them onto the larger landscape organising and containing our daily practice" (Smith, 1987, p. 183). As Greenhalgh (1995) notes, a unified analytical framework fails to depict the complexities of issues on reproductive health. The biosocial framework Jordan (1983) employed in her research captures the intricacies of childbirth practices, but is not adequate enough to understand many pertinent issues. To understand this complexity, a multidimensional framework encompassing culture, gender, socio-economic, political economy and historical perspectives is required.

It is this multidimensional framework, which is central to my analysis, the contention being that the constituting elements of such a framework are critical towards an understanding of childbirth. The framework is organised in terms of the following core themes arising from the results:

- Construction of birth: Limits of plurality;
- Engagement in birthing and embodied knowledge;
- Women's silence: Home and the world;
- Indigenous knowledge of birth: The role of *dainis*;
- Marginalisation of indigenous knowledge;
- Hospital: Power of space and design;
- Authoritative knowledge of biomedical professionals;
- The triad: Doctor, nurse and patient;
- Fiscal Violence; and
- Women, State and obstetric care.

Each theme is separately important to the extent that it illuminates features of birth events. Collectively the themes contribute to an understanding of the social and political constructions of birth in the context of its universal physiological nature. The significance of this analysis lies in exploration of indigenous as well as biomedical knowledge in order to draw out the components of each, thus, enhancing our understanding of childbirth experiences of rural women in Bangladesh.

6.1 CONSTRUCTION OF BIRTH: LIMITS OF PLURALITY

The first reaction of rural women in response to questions on homebirth practices is to ask why, if the baby is born at home normally, should they need to go to the hospital. My analysis of this issue, thus, will address the degree to which childbirth at home is regarded as a normal state as opposed to being difficult. As understanding of childbirth and pregnancy suggests a link with health seeking behaviour (Afsana & Rashid, 2000; Jirojwong, 1996), I will also address how local understanding influences health seeking in birth experiences.

Various 'models' explain pregnancy and birth. The biomedical model, for instance, explains pregnancy and birth as a medical issue. On the other hand, the social model of health considers pregnancy and birth neither as illness nor as sickness (Davis-Floyd, 1992; Kitzinger, 1982; Oakley, 1980; Wagner, 1994). In fact, the social model of health remains very much rooted in Oakley's (1980) classical statement, "Pregnant women are not ill like patients who seek care from hospital for treating illness" (p. 18). The evidence presented in this thesis indicates that, in Bangladesh, rural women's understanding of birth is also located within the social model of health. That is, pregnancy and birth are considered as a "part of daily life" (Wagner, 1994, p. 32) and are, therefore, treated as a normal event. This finding accords with the research amongst the Yucatan and Oaxacan women in Mexico who manage pregnancy and birth within the family or community as a normal event (Jordan, 1983; Sesia, 1997).

The influence of local culture on birthing decisions can be further clarified by contrasting understandings of birth in North American and Bangladeshi societies. According to Davis-Floyd (1992, 1994), North American society itself is responsible for influencing women to behave technocratically and consider birth as a medical event. In brief, birthing practices are shaped by particular discourses produced in what Foucault (as cited in Weedon, 1987) refers to as the "discursive field" (p. 35) consisting of competing ways of giving meaning to the world and of organising social institutions and processes (Weedon, 1987). It is this discourse that produces, accumulates and circulates in a society to give meaning and to influence everyday practices in life (Foucault, 1980a). In non-industrialised, rural Bangladesh, although birth is seen as a normal event, the construction of *thikmoton* (usual) and *kolbekol* (difficult) birth is the result of dominant cultural practices prevailing in the society. On the other hand, in North American society, the recognition of medically assisted vaginal birth as being a normal event is produced by the technocratisation of the society (Davis-Floyd, 1990, 1992, 1994). In North America, this happens because the core cultural value system is developed on a paradigm of science, technology, patriarchy and institutions (Davis-Floyd, 1992; Reynolds, 1991), whereas in rural Bangladesh social values developed from daily life and social realities are practically devoid of scientific and technological influence. This contrasting approach to life offers critical implications for birthing in Bangladesh.

Knowledge, as generally held, is constructed from life circumstances and experiences (Foster & Anderson, 1978). It is in this context that Kleinman (1986) argues that the meaning of illness is constructed by everyday experiences – "the way the sick person and the members of her or his social network come to perceive, live with and respond to symptoms" (p. 151). Similarly, women's meanings of birth are shaped by their personal and circumstantial experiences. Put slightly differently, women's construction of birth is not only shaped by the birth experiences of women but also influenced by the context in which the meaning of birth is produced. In fact, the meaning of *thikmoton* and *kolbekol* birth is constructed in the light of similarity or dissimilarity to other births regularly occurring in the village. The understanding here corresponds to what Derrida meant by *différance*, that is, the meaning is produced through dual strategies of difference and deferral (Weedon, 1987). Rural women's understanding of birth as *thikmoton* and *kolbekol* is produced with differences and deferral in the meaning of birth in the village of Bangladesh. The strategies employed in managing birth are influenced by the paradigm of meaning and also how others in the family or society behave in the task of helping women give birth.

It is important not to dichotomise understandings of birth and position them simply at two extremes. Although birth is centered on *thikmoton* and *kolbekol*, there are various experiences that persist across this dichotomy and impart plurality to the meaning of birth. The demarcation of birth events is otherwise far from being rigid and fixed, there is considerable overlapping due to the unfixed, plural meaning of birth. It is this unfixed meaning of birth that gives rise to a situation where the paradigm of *thikmoton* includes births that are managed in home but requires medical assistance. The delivery of breech presentation or contracted pelvis regularly occurs in home amidst the presence of *dainis* and the use of "simultaneous resorts" (Kleinman, 1980, p. 187), such as amulets, sanctified water and herbal roots used for supernatural causalities and bodily imbalance. These prevailing practices persuade others to adopt similar measures, which are observed in everyday practices in the village. The understandings of birth developed within the socio-cultural context make people undecided about seeking emergency obstetric care. At times, this brings sufferings to rural women's birth experiences. In this context, Jordan (1983) argues, "Discrepancies between the local and the medical definition militate against the utilisation of the resources of hospital obstetrics even for the cases that clearly fall into the medical realm" (p. 79).

The meaning of birth and the strategies adopted to cope with the birth crisis are constructed by the understandings produced within the social context. In the Western world, debate continues between the social and medical models of defining pregnancy and childbirth as being either a natural or medical event. What is constituted in this definition of birth influences women's choice of care, but it neither affects their health seeking behaviour nor impedes their access to obstetric facilities irrespective of their proclivity to natural or biomedical model of birthing. In rural Bangladesh, however, women's health care seeking is very much influenced by the plural meanings of birth, floating between *thikmoton* and *kolbekol*. These women have neither choice of care nor adequate access to obstetric facilities. What happens is that when the normal event of birth hits complications, their access to obstetric care is affected by the socially constructed meaning of birth that, at times, can prove fatal both to the mother and the child.

6.2 EMBODIED KNOWLEDGE AND ENGAGEMENT IN BIRTH

Rural women actively participate and engage themselves in birth events. To understand the process, an analysis is done on how women draw on their knowledge to actively engage or disengage in the events. I argue how mind-body integration, embodied knowledge and shared knowledge are constructed facilitating women's active involvement in birth.

Integration of mind and body is assured in a holistic or midwifery, or social models of birth (Dais-Floyd, 1992, 1994; Rothman, 1982). Contrasting childbirth from the context of biomedical and midwifery models, Rothman (1982) states, "the latter is based on an integration of mind and body so that physical events can be seen as socially done" (p. 181). She argues that where birthing women adopt an active role, the syncretisation of mind and body is crucial for participation in the birth experience. Davis-Floyd (1992) expresses similar views of mind and body integration from the holistic ideology of home-birthers in the USA. In rural, birth settings of Bangladesh, women's articulation of the collective influence of *moner shahosh* (mental strength) and *shoriler shakti* (physical strength) is the expression of uniting mind and body as an individual unit. Women consider the importance of harmonious coordination between mind and body in giving birth. It is this knowledge that is constructed by women from their personal and circumstantial experiences bringing confidence in their active participation of birth.

Different views exist about the act of mind and body. In *Spiritual Midwifery*, a midwife comments, "Since body and mind are one, sometimes you can fix the mind by working on the body, and you can fix the body by working on the mind" (Gaskin, 1990, p. 344). The argument of Davis-Floyd (1992) and Cosslett (1994) is based on the holistic paradigm where they claim that mind and body are one and interconnected. Rural women in Bangladesh treat mind and body as separate entities, but insist on their living in harmonious relationship. The feeble engagement of mind and body in birth experiences may result in their disconnectedness and lead to unsuccessful birth. As such, malnourishment and older age are considered bodily unfit for participating in birth events, whereas first-time mother and educated women are seen as mentally not strong in facing birth experience. Different approaches are, therefore, employed by rural women to strengthen the role of mind and body, which leads to their interconnected harmony in achieving successful birth.

The holistic, midwifery, or indigenous model, whatever term is used, opposes the views of the medical or technocratic model that underpins the Cartesian split between mind and body. This was first developed in the philosophy of René Descartes (1596-1650) where the body is seen as a mechanical metaphor giving supremacy to mind over body (Lock & Scheper-Hughes, 1990; Rothman, 1982). In extending the Cartesian legacy, Lock and Scheper-Hughes (1990) argue, "The higher 'essence' of man, the rational mind, was thus extracted from nature, allowing a rigorous objective examination of nature, including human body, for the first time in Western history" (p. 52). As such, in the hospitals of Bangladesh, strict confinement to bed and manoeuvring and mutilation of the body enable biomedical professionals to take control over birth events. This scenario is portrayed in Rothman's (1982) description of hospital birth, "The birth is managed, conducted, by the other members of the team, those who are telling her what to do, and physically manipulating her and her baby" (p. 177). As body is the centre of attention, mind is totally being ignored by the lack of emotional support and the intimidating attitudes of doctors and nurses resulting in psychological sufferings and isolation of rural women. The disconnectedness of mind and body is the result of "failure to conceptualise a mindful causation of somatic states" (Lock & Scheper-Hughes, 1990, p. 52). In this medical mode, the body-centric management and the psychological isolation eventually dislocate rural women from their own birth experience.

The Cartesian concept of the mind's supremacy over the body prevails among women in the technocratised society of USA (Cranny-

Francis, 1995; Davis-Floyd, 1992, 1994). Unlike biomedical perspectives, Bangladeshi, rural women's view about mind and body is not based on the supremacy of mind over body. The relationship of physical and psychological experiences is articulated in women's voice as interdependent. They stress that mind and body act as mutually dependent, separateness of one fails to accomplish the errand of achieving birth.

The understanding of bodily experiences influences women to actively participate in birth. Davis-Floyd (1994) denotes it as an inner knowing or women's intuition, which is an important characteristic of holistic models of birth. Graham and Oakley (1981) claim that this knowledge is women's own capacity to sense and react to the sensations of their body. They (1981) also argue, "It is thus an individualised and to some extent intuitive knowledge built up from bodily experiences" (p. 55). This argument underpins the view that women's active participation of birth is made possible through inner knowing of body (Davis-Floyd, 1992). Yet, this inner knowing is socially constructed created from women's personal and shared experiences that become embodied. It is understood from the birth event of the first-time mother, who lacks this inner knowing, as opposed to birth event of experienced mother. On the other hand, in hospital birth, the passivity of women may result from a lack of inner knowing especially among formally educated women who may only experience hospital or nurse assisted birth, and from authoritarian environment, non-supportive of women with inner knowledge. The socially constructed knowledge of inner knowing interconnected with bodily mechanisms leads women to actively engage in achieving birth.

The harmonious connectedness between mind and body and understanding of bodily mechanisms are intensified by the synchronised cooperation of all other women participating in a birth event. In the midwifery model, birthing women are given the central role, but the event is accomplished by the participation of other women who engage their mind and body in its success (Rothman, 1982). These women share their bodily experiences by telling stories and providing emotional supports that emphasise the unity of mind and body. Like Jordan (1983), I also claim that birth is a communal or collective event in which *dainis* or *parteras* and many other women participate together sharing their knowledge and experiences to support birthing women physically and emotionally. Jordan (1997) refers to this as authoritative knowledge defined as consensually constructed and socially produced. Each woman participating in birth owns, reproduces and reinforces this knowledge (Jordan, 1983; Sesia, 1997). The findings of my research accord with Jordan's description of women's participation where all the women become active participants in birth. Nevertheless, I prefer to use collective or shared or communal knowledge rather than authoritative knowledge. The very word 'authoritative' conveys a message of dominance, which seems to be lacking in birth events that I have described. Although, *dainis* are more experienced and skilled than others, all the participants remain as mutual exchangers of knowledge in the birth event.

Kitzinger (1991, 2002) stresses the importance of women's supportive roles that give strength and confidence to birthing women. Jordan (1983) describes this support system lacking in hospital birth as,

> The interactional environment in the hospital is fundamentally different from the home environment not only by virtue of the absence of familiar resources of psychological support for the mother, but also by virtue of the presence of the medical delivery team whose members are inappropriate birth attendants by the standards of the indigenous system. (p. 84)

In the Bangladeshi hospitals, women not only lack emotional support, but also endure emotional abuse in medical encounters causing demoralisation and loss of self-confidence. Yet, an informal system of emotional support is created by the involvement of a special *ayah*, who forcefully attends birth out of economic necessity, and a woman family member who is allowed to stay close to birthing woman during birth event. In spite of the dominant authoritarian bio-medical control, a more supportive environment is created in labour room not through proper planning but due to shortage of medical personnel in hospital.

The sharing of knowledge is supported by Irigaray's (1991) views of woman-to-woman sociality, which eventually create the personal and collective identity of women. In relation to improving women's mental and emotional health, the approach of story telling and women-to-women support were also observed in Hunt's (1998) research. This approach is employed in self-help groups[1] developed in the women's health movement (Broom, 1991; Doyal, 1995). Sharing knowledge is, in fact, a self-help approach, developed in this village within women's domain, but without any visible movement. This shared knowledge gives rural women a specific identity where their knowledge is created, circulated and generated in a critical, joyful moment of life during childbirth.

The significance of this knowledge is obvious when rural women manage birth in their own terrain; the unification of mind/body, understandings of bodily experiences and the necessity of shared knowledge are crucial in birth event. This knowledge is also important, as women give birth with uncertain consequences. As Fromm (1955) states, each step into a different, human existence is frightening because it is new and unknown. In this situation, women consider that disharmony of this knowledge impedes the usual process of birth, and if problems arise it cannot be resolved within their own domain of knowledge. However, the uncertainty of birth consequences widens the plurality of understandings and eventually leads them to search for different options of care. Nandy (1995) argues on the strength of scepticism in traditional medicine as opposed to modern biomedicine where there is no space left for self-doubt and self-criticism and for seeking other options. Scepticism, in fact, opens up the space for rectification and improvement of the existing practices and at the same time, acknowledges the existence of other birthing care. The embodied knowledge enables women to actively engage in birth event, but scepticism in birth consequences leads them to search for other options of care.

6.3 WOMEN'S SILENCE: HOME AND THE WORLD

Rural women are silent while giving birth at home or in hospital. At home observance of silence in pregnancy and childbirth is rooted in *sharam*, a social attribute expected in women's character. In explication of women's sufferings in South Asia, Ahmed (1999) claims that women's silence is influenced by feminine principles intrinsic in Indian religious and mythological Goddesses. Partha Chatterjee (1993) elucidates the feminine quality drawing on Bengali middle class women in colonial and post-colonial Indian State. This author claims that the new construct of fernity based on the spiritual qualities of self-sacrifice, benevolence, devotion, religiosity, modesty, tolerance and so on is inherent in the indigenous social roles of women buttressed by the force of mythological inspirations. Rural women's *sharam* is nothing but an extension of modesty and other qualities expected in the indigenous feminine character. Because of *sharam*, the news of conception is kept silent and secret, birth events are observed secretly and labour pain is endured silently. This unexpressed expression of silence is a socially obligated burden, which rural women carry on for years and for which they also suffer. In *History of Sexuality*, Foucault (1978) associates silence, secrecy and tolerance with prohibitory sexual practices. In *Apurbabari* village, birth is not a prohibited matter, but *sharam*, tolerance and silence act as prohibitory social practices making women suffer silently. As a consequence, serious pregnancy and birth-related crisis may occasionally remain unnoticed, unacknowledged that prevents women from seeking necessary and appropriate care.

Women's silence in birth event varies with experience and age. Studies in many other parts of India document the observance of silence in birth events. Of particular note is a study done in two villages of North India by Jeffery, Jeffery and Lyon (1989). They try to associate silence with *sharam*, but I disagree with the authors' constant use of the word – shame for '*sharam*' denoting shameful, immodest behaviour. Their analysis of silence and *sharam* is based on the women's low status in India rather than the indigenous feminine principle discussed above. The definition of status is a very complex issue in South Asia. The status of women is not a direct expression of difference from men. In Indian society, women's status varies with the different stages of life cycle revealing a very influential relationship with their sons (Nandy, 1990). With increasing age, experience and motherhood women secure higher status in their home domain. Patel (1999) argues that with increasing age and number of children, women attain positions to influence decisions on fertility behaviour without ousting mothering and patriarchy. In a rural family, in the context of birth, all women regardless of their age and experience remain silent. Experienced women are expected to be more tolerant and silent in birth than women with no experience. In this context, silence does not indicate a status differential among women themselves. Nevertheless, all the women equally become victim of the feminine characteristics burdened with silence.

Weedon's (1987) argument, developed from Foucauldian perspectives, supports the gendered constitution of silence locating its origin in patriarchal subjection of power. Chatterjee (1993) claims that the feminine quality maintained in the inner world – 'home' is the result of traditional Indian patriarchy.[2] Bordo (1999), on the other hand, argues that in modern Western society, normative feminine practices produced and reproduced in cultural demands give rise to docility and obedience in female body. It is this docility and subservience to normative feminine practices that account for rural women's silence in pregnancy and birth. The maintenance of feminine qualities is described as subjectivity, which is referred to as, "conscious and unconscious thoughts and emotions of the individual, her sense of herself and her ways of understanding her relation to the world" (Weedon, 1987, p. 32). In the rural context, the constitution of women's subjectivity produced within the discursive practices of Indian traditional patriarchy makes women docile and thus, silent, tolerant and modest. The feminine qualities of powerful Indian Goddesses are essentially intended for the emancipation not for the repression of women. But, in cultural practices, these qualities now serve to keep rural women's sufferings in silence.

While giving birth in hospital rural women become quiet and silent. Giving birth in a hospital reduces women to patient status (Rothman, 1982). In *The Oxford Illustrated Dictionary* (Coulson, Carr, Hutchison & Eagle, 1962), the word 'patient' means one having patience or a person under medical treatment, especially with reference to his doctor. In a medical establishment, women are transformed into patients through multiple rituals of medicalised treatment (Martin, 1989; Oakley 1980; Rothman 1982). Yet, the very meaning of the word, 'patience' that carries a sense of being quiet and acquiescent is applicable to rural women when they undergo hospital birth in Bangladesh. Biomedical models of treatment based on scientific and rationalistic, modern, Western patriarchy (Good, 1997) create male-centric management in Bangladeshi hospital obstetric facilities even with the preponderance of female health providers. Under these circumstances, the medicalised experience of birth and unusual experiences in the hospital reinforce rural women's patience and silence.

Women's silence is expressed in their disciplining and conformity to medical authority. The disciplining of patients is caused by "bio-power" in which numerous and diverse techniques are employed "for achieving the subjugation of bodies and the control of populations" (Foucault, 1978, p. 140). The body becomes the place of contestations of power to make patients disciplined and self-regulating – "docile" bodies (Foucault, 1978). As a consequence, rural women silently conform to the authority of doctors and nurses. Bartky (1986, as cited in Sawicki, 1991) argues, from Foucauldian perspectives that the silencing and powerlessness result from disciplining of the feminine body. This silencing and powerlessness cause rural women to suffer physically as well as emotionally. As Foucault (1978) reasons, where there is power, there is resistance. Women's silence does not indicate agreement with everything rather it is expressed as resistance against the medicalised experiences, the authority of biomedical professionals and unfamiliar situation in the hospital. Women are made silent by the disciplining power of cosmopolitan obstetrics, but they remain silent by manipulating resistance in the form of non-cooperation and denial to accept their care. Within women's silence, both power and resistance are displayed. Silence is, therefore, approved as a mark of discipline, but resentment is expressed within silence. Rural, poor women simultaneously conform to and deny the authority of cosmopolitan obstetrics.

Women's silence in birth causes sufferings, no matter where the birth occurs. At home, rural women are subjected to silence by their intrinsic feminine qualities. On the other hand, in hospital, the imposed patient role objectifies women to remain silent through disciplining of the body. Yet their resistance intensifies this silence. As Das (1997) states, "Tradition is what diminishes women and permits a subtle everyday violence to be perpetrated upon them" (p. 75). In this context, rural women's sufferings in silence are tantamount to violence perpetrated by the traditional value system. This exposition of violence goes beyond tradition when she observes violence in modernity, as it is reflected in women's silence and sufferings in hospital birth. Standing on the brink of modern society, traditional, rural women suffer as victim of both traditional values and modern technological system.

6.4 INDIGENOUS KNOWLEDGE OF BIRTH: THE ROLE OF *DAINIS*

In most developing countries, childbirth still depends on indigenous knowledge of birth where traditional midwives play a special role (Afsana & Rashid, 2000; Blanchet, 1984; Chawla, 2002; Cosminsky, 1982; Jeffery, Jeffery & Lyon, 1989; Jordan, 1983; Kay, 1982; Kitzinger, 1982; Laderman, 1982; MacCormack, 1982; Ram, 2001; Rozario, 1998; Sargent, 1982; Unnithan-Kumar, 2002). Conflicting views of midwives regarding their expertise, role and status have been observed cross-culturally. Despite midwives' expertise in attending normal deliveries, most research highlight their lack of skills in managing complicated cases. The sole supportive role of midwives is debated, as birth is accomplished in the presence of other women and, in some cultures, husbands or fathers also take part. In some societies, the high status of midwives is observed in their caring role before and after the birth event. Research findings in Bangladesh and India offer contrasting views where some studies confer low status to midwives while others suggest that midwives are respected and held a high status in their own community. In many parts of Bangladesh, *dainis* are called as *dhoruni* – baby catcher indicating their unimportant role in birth events (Blanchet, 1984; Rozario, 1995). Although, *dhoruni* is seldom used in *Apurbabari* village, I argue that when birthing women are expected to play an active role, *dainis'* role should not be more than a *dhoruni*. In reality, *dainis* play more of a role than a baby catcher. *Daini's* expertise, role and status must be explicated to understand why rural women still count on *dainis* as their birth attendant.

A considerable body of research acknowledges indigenous expertise, but little is documented about what actually happens. Jordan (1983) offers a valuable account of indigenous skills among Mayan midwives, but also draws attention to practices that are futile or even deleterious to the progress of labour. Similarly, many useful skills of traditional midwives are observed in Kay (1982) and Kitzinger's (1991) research on birth practices. The present study also shows that many of *dainis' skills* are practical, useful facilitating the process of birth. It includes non-restriction of movement, intermittent walking and resting, holding onto a bamboo pole or rope, taking on different postures, self-evacuation of bladder and bowel, non-interference in actual birthing, and methods employed for perineal protection and placental expulsion. Similar practices observed in birth events across cultures are considered useful by many experts (Cosminsky, 1982; Jordan, 1983; Kay, 1982; Kitzinger, 1991). Squeezing umbilical cord to pull blood is regularly practiced but is disputed in medical practice, as it may cause occasional rise of blood volume in premature neonates. Kitzinger (1981) suggests in her manual on homebirth that women should continue eating that acts as an energiser. In indigenous birth practices, women are served warm rice and encouraged to drink water or milk. Warm compression applied over the perineum improves healing process, quickens uterine involution and gives comfort to birthing women. These practices are also documented in Belle's (2002) cross-cultural research in India and Japan. For natural post-partum bleeding, frequent change of petticoats seems more useful than wearing ragged clothes especially for the purpose of reducing puerperal infections. This indigenous knowledge of birth and associated practices remain unheeded due to lack of comparative analysis with other indigenous birthing cultures and hospital birth practices.

Explications of touch in diverse cultures draw attention to the contrasting practices between indigenous birth and cosmopolitan obstetrics (Kitzinger, 1997). Touching birthing women's body is "one way of knowing" (Kitzinger, 1997, p. 209), which *dainis* essentially perform in indigenous birthing. Different touches, such as blessings, comforting, physical support, diagnosis and even punitive are carried out in different forms in birth practices. In birth events, massaging oil on the birthing women's head and abdomen, shaking waist and lubricating perineal area with oil are commonly performed by *dainis* to ease the process of birthing whereas other women partook by pressing limbs and embracing birthing women. Kitzinger (1997) claims that this touch has a great impact in enhancing woman-to-woman sociality, giving confidence to women, easing the birth process and contributing to reduction of complications. On the other hand, touch is expressed as restraining or punitive (Kitzinger, 1997), as it happens in the hospitals of Bangladesh when doctors and nurses restrict women's movement and disgrace them with verbal and occasional physical abuse. This feeling gives rise to a desolate experience where women feel victimised, violated and invaded, which Kitzinger (1997) denotes as "violence against women" (p. 229).

Practices identified as harmful in TBA training programmes are continually observed regardless of their training status (Goodburn et al., 1994; Goodburn, Chowdhury, Gazi, Marshall & Graham, 2000; Akhter, Rahman, Mannan, Elahi & Khan, 1995). In my observation, nearly all *dainis* did not wash their hands before touching the birth canal in spite of their awareness of 'three cleans': clean hands, clean blades and clean areas. The reason for using unwashed hands is that vaginal blood is considered as unclean and polluting. Thus, hand washing with water is performed subsequent to touching birth canal in order to remove impurity, which is also observed by Blanchet (1984) and Rozario (1998) in their research conducted elsewhere in Bangladesh. Moreover, notions of germ and infections do not exist in people's mind. Concurrently, in a poor house, soap is a luxury item used economically and cautiously. When *dainis* are constantly accused of causing puerperal infections due to their unhygienic birth practices (Blanchet, 1984), research in Bangladesh shows that puerperal infections are not related to the 'three cleans' as taught by WHO but to malnutrition and living conditions (Goodburn, et al., 2000). *Dainis'* interventions become harmful when birth becomes complicated. Despite their understanding that frequent touching is a bad practice, the birth canal is undoubtedly manipulated when *dainis* fail to manage birth. A difficult birth creates panic, and therefore, its management is carried out through the interventions of several *dainis*. This causes harm to mother and foetus due to frequent handling and forceful delivery. It is crucial to consider these issues. Some maternal and child deaths and morbidities can be minimised if *dainis* do not further intervene because the knowledge and skills required to manage birth complications do not fall within their domain of knowledge.

Many obstetric practices in Bangladeshi hospitals are antagonistic to indigenous birth practices. Frequent touching of the birth canal is considered to be badly reputed *daini's* practice in *Apurbabari* village, but is a common event observed in the study hospitals. Frequent handling of birth canal increases the risk of infections (Kitzinger, 1997). It is reported that the number of vaginal examinations in a birth event is directly related to puerperal infections, not the length of time after the rupture of the membrane (Wagner, Chin, Peters, Drexler & Newman, 1989). What surprised me most is that doctors and nurses, trained in theories of germs and infections, invariably use non-sterilised instruments, gloves and syringe needles. Jordan (1983) refers to this as "doing scientific obstetrics badly" (p. 77). One study in India reveals that the infection rate for child deliveries in hospital is 23 percent, whereas it is five percent at home (Bajpai, 1996, as cited in Belle 2002). This study suggests that the risk of infection is likely to be high in the hospital as opposed to home due to unhygienic practices and cross-infections. The frightening issue is that medical personnel are knowingly doing bad scientific obstetric practices.

Emotional and physical support is essential during childbirth. According to Trevanthan (1997), "Birth is such a powerful emotional as well as physical experience for all women is that it is these emotions (e.g., fear, anxiety, uncertainty) that lead them to seek assistance, whereby mortality is reduced" (p. 84). Although this argument is specifically founded on evolutionary perspectives of birthing, it supports the fact that companionship is critical in birth events. Cosminsky (1982) confirms this analysis noting that the "Traditional role is an expanded role, part of the support system includes social, ritual and psychological components" (p. 217). She underscores the importance of support systems in indigenous birth practices. In similar vein, traditional midwives and the other women are seen to offer emotional and physical supports in indigenous birthing across cultures (Jordan, 1983; Rothman, 1982; Kitzinger, 1997), which are also predominantly observed in *Apurbabari* village. In birth events, even with their experience and skills, *dainis* try not to domineer birthing women, but to open a space where birthing women play a pivotal role. Mutual communications of birth experiences, sharing of knowledge and continual encouragement create a horizontal, non-hierarchical relationship where women gain confidence to achieve a successful birth outcome. *Dainis'* supporting role is expressed in their voice, touch and rituals in assisting women to achieve birth. The physical contact and emotional attachment make their involvement significant in each birth event. This is an important issue, which indicates why doctors and nurses in the hospital and male *dai* from their own community cannot become integral partners in the event. Moreover, despite abusive criticisms of doctors and nurses, *dainis'* supportive roles are observed in hospitals accompanying birthing women. No bio-medical professionals would expect to be recognised as supportive as *dainis* to birthing women.

In indigenous birth practices of other cultures, the selection of midwives begins in their early interactions with women in antenatal care (Jordan, 1983, Kitzinger, 1982; Laderman, 1982). Even in cosmopolitan obstetrics, except for public services, midwives or obstetrician are selected in a similar fashion (Davis-Floyd, 1992; Jordan, 1983). The relationship between women and birth attendants is developed in antenatal period where respectful attitudes and trust grow between them. In contrast, in *Apurbabari*, as antenatal care does not exist in indigenous birth practices, interactions with *dainis* and the development of relationships happen differently. As Kakar (1980) emphasises, trust and dependence on *dais* have grown through ages in rural societies in India. In *Apurbabari*, the *dainis'* selection depends on the familial relationship with women as well as their trust in them. People are aware of who are the skilled and experienced *dainis* in the village, but trust is not built on their special expertise. Successful and satisfactory assistance in previous family births and maintenance of privacy develop trust and dependence on *dainis*. The practicality of seeking kin *dainis* is that most live within the family boundary. Yet, trust is so important that *dainis* living afar are fetched secretly without drawing public notice. Privacy is infringed when someone outside the domain of family is contacted. A nurse-attended birth event is considered as a violation of privacy, as it is exposed to the outside world. To maintain silence and privacy, I was not called in by a family in a birth event, even with my professional degrees and with my close relationship with them. Later on, I understood that I was not able to gain their sufficient trust to attend such a private, familial event. Hence, trust and dependence developed on long-term interactions are deemed essential for attending indigenous birth in *Apurbabari* village rather than specialised skills or expertise of birth attendants.

A considerable amount of research suggests that the social position of *dais* is seen lowly because their task is associated with touching and removing birth pollution – a menial job in society (Blanchet, 1984; Rozario, 1995, 1998; Jeffery, Jeffery & Lyon, 1989). Not only is the status of the job low, it is also intensified by the poor-socio-economic status of *dainis* and women's low status in the society. Their argument is the result of modern political discourse, which is based on rationality, capitalism and institutions. However, this argument essentialises the variety of birth experiences as revealed in my research of a *daini's* position in a poor, Muslim society. Firstly, in a village such as *Apurbabari*, everyone is economically poor. As such, a *daini* is not singled-out as a poor individual. Secondly, as childbirth is a women's domain, a *daini* as a wise woman is not affected by women's low status due to her experience and age. Thirdly, a *daini* accepts this 'lowly, polluted' task willingly to meet the practical needs of women, but not to satisfy the economic necessity. More importantly, the fixity of meaning given to pollution in language does not remain so in lived experience, which is reflected in birthing women's behaviour in not strictly observing pollution rituals in the seclusion period. It is this modern discourse that insists on fixed, determinate, form of meanings ignoring the human priorities produced in contextuality (Chatterjee, 1993). The meaning of pollution is more significant in the Brahminical value systems than in a poor, low caste. In *Apurbabari,* women with skills of *daini* are not considered socially degraded. Rather they earn a respectable position in their own society. Kakar (1980) also observes that in Hindu society, *dais* earn trust and confidence among their own people. The problem of *dais'* status is not associated with birth pollution rather with the valuation of jobs produced by social stratification and monetary values given to the task. The task is not seen as polluted, when women of well-off families perform *dai's* task in their own families as well as in poor families, nurses attend birth within or outside hospital regardless of classes, and upper class women become obstetricians. This analysis is supported by Somjee's (1991) argument that doctor's profession is not seen as polluting as it was in ancient time. He (1991) continues to argue that doctors are now treated as if they come from higher Brahminic caste because the modern capitalistic society adds monetary values to their status. The stink of pollution is, therefore, removed with the valuation of job. My argument is that the low status of a *dai* is not produced within her own society but by the Brahminical values of caste system and by the modern capitalist society conferring a particular monetary value to her task.

Dainis remain as traditional midwives in *Apurbabari,* but do not take midwifery as an occupation. It is stated in the dictionary entry on childbirth of *Blackwell Dictionary of Anthropology* (Barfield, 1996) that in the Islamic society of Bangladesh, the midwifery tradition did not develop due to its association with birth pollution. As an outcome of the present study, I argue that midwives always exist in this society to meet the needs of women during and, at times, after the birth event. Yet, they are not established as an occupation like traditional midwives in other societies. As midwifery is a communal knowledge, all women are expected to have some knowledge in managing birth. More importantly, notions of purdah impede the development of midwifery as an occupation in Muslim peasant society. Women's movements are limited to their family domain due to existing practices of purdah. This makes midwifery unappealing because, within family boundaries, pecuniary gain is nil or minimum. The evidence in this study indicated that remunerating *daini's* with cash is not customary in rural society.[3] Chawla (2002) confirms that as *dais'* work is an extension of women's work, the traditional *jajmani* system is operated through the exchange of goods for services. Thus, even if *dainis* work outside their family domain, their services may not be reimbursed in cash. Within the family domain, the role of *daini* remains within the pre-capitalist, pre-modern societal value system where their work value is associated more with earning mental and spiritual satisfaction than with monetary value. But, in this poverty-stricken society that has become entrenched with the modern capitalist development, *dainis* would be caught in further poverty if they relied on midwifery as their only occupation.

Indigenous birth is based on communal knowledge continually produced and reproduced by personal, circumstantial and experiential experiences of women. The *dainis'* role remains significant not only for possessing knowledge in managing birth, but also in providing support to birthing women. Yet, in a difficult birth, the whole domain of indigenous knowledge becomes handicapped, because it has been neglected and under-researched for the possibilities it can offer. It is this issue of the marginalisation of indigenous knowledge that provides the focus of the next section.

6.5 MARGINALISATION OF INDIGENOUS KNOWLEDGE

Indigenous knowledge of birth is in danger of being dislocated by the upsurge of modern biomedicine (Davis-Floyd & Sargent, 1997). The central contention is that technomedical systems relying on science and technology replace indigenous systems of birth. It is in this context, Chawla (2002) argues, that not only is indigenous knowledge marginalised, but also is poor, rural women who own this knowledge. In different cultures, marginalised groups, such as sorcerers and witches are identified as source of dangers doing harm (Favre-Saada, 1980; Lindenbaum, 1979). The rationality of modern medicine identifies traditional midwives as a potential source of danger causing harm to the society (Ram, 2001). Ram (2001) also reasons that the technicality of biomedicine displaces knowledge from women's domain giving rise to mechanistic knowledge of birth. However, Chawla (2002) argues that the disregard for traditional midwives is the result of colonial devaluation of indigenous knowledge of birth practices. In this vein of discussion, Ram (2001) suggests that it is the multiple modernities, that is, colonial force and biomedical expansion that cause traditional midwives to become the victims of contested territory of childbirth assistance. This analysis accords with the literatures that focus on colonialism, modernity and biomedicine as sources of the marginalisation of indigenous knowledge of birth. Let me explain how indigenous knowledge of *dainis* is marginalised in Bangladesh.

Traditional midwives' knowledge in ancient India was challenged during the colonial period. In ancient India, *dais* were considered as the birth attendants, as they played a much wider role including lay gynaecologists, herbalists, nutritionists and psychiatrists caring for the health problems of rural women (Kakar, 1980). *Dais'* skills were recognised both in lower and upper caste society despite the fact that *dais* were members of untouchable castes (Somjee, 1991). In colonial India, these social relationships started to change. The colonisers had contempt for indigenous practices and sought to abolish Ayurvedic practices (Gupta, 1976). Indigenous midwives were caught in this 'eye' of contempt. As Ram (2001) argues, "what was at stake in India was not a simple project of modernity as a reform, but reform as redefined by the politics of colonialism itself" (p. 66). What she is suggesting is that the interplay of colonialism and modernity invades indigenous culture by questioning the scientific principle of childbirth practices. The white women doctors who were marginalised in their own society came to displace local midwives in India. These lady doctors were primarily urban and missionary based. *Dai* practices were highly criticised for the lack of hygienic standards decided by the missionaries and white woman doctors (Somjee, 1991; Shetty, 1994 as cited in Ram, 2001). In 1860, *dai* training first started in India and was reinvented every 20 years thereafter (Jeffery, Jeffery & Lyon, 1989). For more than a century, lessons from the previous training were never taken into account for the next. In time, *dais* were left to attend to poor, rural women, whilst Indian, middle class women took the place of the white lady doctor (Ram, 2001).

The Traditional Birth Attendant (TBA) training programme is a new initiative in an attempt to biomedicalise *dainis'* knowledge. To ensure safe delivery, discourses on TBA training began throughout the developing world with the Safe Motherhood Initiatives of World Health Organisation and UNICEF. In Bangladesh, under the Directorate of Family Planning, a nationwide TBA training programme began in 1979 to improve maternal and child health.[4] The introduction of new knowledge was initiated, which was completely biomedicine-centric. This didactic, formal approach essentially sought to institute hygienic birth practices and to encourage referral of complicated pregnancies to hospital. In the mid-nineties, TBA training was discontinued because the programme did not seem to improve their performance (Ministry of Health and Family Welfare, 1998a). Failure of the programme is blamed on TBAs for not incorporating biomedical knowledge into their own practices. Until recently, mismanaged training and supervision of trained TBAs were not documented. However, research in Mexico demonstrates the continuing gulf between indigenous knowledge and TBA training lessons (Jordan, 1989). The way of transferring knowledge and, more importantly, the complete exclusion of indigenous knowledge (Jordan, 1989) doom such training to failure. In this context, Jordan (1989) argues, "cosmopolitan obstetrics becomes a cosmopolitical obstetrics, that is to say, a system which enforces a particular distribution of power across cultural and social divisions" (p. 935). This means that the promotion of medicalised training courses as the only legitimate knowledge implicitly devalues local knowledge and outlaws indigenous skills acquisition. In the Bangladeshi context, the failure of TBA programmes is also the result of the medicalised content and didactic training from which *dainis'* worldviews of birth and their ways of learning are diametrically opposed. Ram (2001), on the other hand, claims that the medicalised training of TBAs is an attempt to use *dais* as 'intermediary' to serve the biomedical practitioners. In fact, this intermediary role of dais or *dainis* was observed in colonised India to serve lady doctors (Ram, 2001), in India to refer family planning patients to health centres (Jeffery, Jeffery & Lyon, 1989) and in Bangladesh to send high 'risk' pregnancies to hospitals (Akhter et al., 1995) to benefit the bio-medical practitioners.

In the contestations of colonialism, modernity and biomedicine, the indigenous knowledge of *dainis* is continually challenged. The colonial invasion of the Westerners into India sought to destroy the indigenous practices of *dais*. In the 21st century, the TBA-training programme is a neo-colonial invasion of biomedicine intending to abolish indigenous knowledge of *daini,* akin to the witch-hunts carried out during the medieval period in Europe (Ehrenreich & English 1973). In recent times, the *dainis'* knowledge in the eyes of the 'enlightened' world turns into vacuity. Abusive criticisms and disapproval of *dainis'* knowledge by biomedical practitioners and the distrust of modern educated women are the public face of this contestation. Yet, the indigenous knowledge of *dainis* survives in its own term in their own community within the domain of home where world-views of birth, life and death are shared. On the other hand, in the external world, they question the legitimacy of their experiential knowledge as opposed to doctors' 'bookish' knowledge. *Dainis* are themselves caught in the web of modernity forfeiting their own expertise to the authoritarian knowledge of biomedicine by being sceptical of their own.

6.6 HOSPITAL: POWER OF DESIGN AND SPACE

Rural women seek refuge in hospital obstetric care, particularly during birth complications. Nevertheless, hospital is the place that creates fear among women. The word hospital derives from the Latin adjective 'hospitalis' which refers to 'hospites' or guests (Turner, 1987). The original meaning of the term is preserved in the notion of hospitality. Whatever is the meaning and intention of the word, the hospitals in Bangladesh carry a sense of fear for rural women and their families. My analysis proceeds with how the design, spatial distribution of hospitals and urbanism make rural, poor women hesitate to seek cosmopolitan obstetric care.

The structural design of hospital buildings is indifferent to the expectations and surroundings known to rural, poor women. Within the enormity of the hospital building women not only misplace them, but also encounter predicaments at each step of their movement as a result of its organisation and the decorum of communications. In *The*

Birth of the Clinic Foucault (1973) argues that the colossal dimension of the hospital edifice is intended to accommodate diverse categories of patients for the beneficence of doctors. The disciplinary power embedded in the *"techne"* (Foucault, 1987a, p. 255) of architecture is what Foucault (1982a) terms, "Bentham's Panopticon" (p. 191), meant for the surveillance of patients and treatment of diseases in hospitals. In this context, I may argue that in Bangladesh, the architectural design and spatial configuration of hospitals are convenient for training doctors, monitoring patients and curing diseases. Yet, what is apposite for learning and curing creates fear and insecurity among poor, illiterate, rural women due to its unfamiliar, socially distant situations.

The hospital building itself stands with its own glory and authority in Bangladesh. Not only the power in *techne* is displayed in spatial configuration, but the architectural design itself also reveals the power struggles, identity and material culture of society (Lawrence, 1992; Vivoni-Farge, 2002). Their central argument is that all the buildings are the products of social and cultural conditions that denote political power in pluralistic societies. Turner (1987), on the other hand, reasons that the growing status and prestige of medical professions given rise to the modern hospital system are reflected in the massive architecture of hospital building. It is in this context, I shall argue that the massiveness of the hospital building symbolises the authoritarian status of the government, and the social status of modern biomedical professionals, but to the detriment of poor, rural women who get perplexed within the puzzles of hospital buildings. These poor women lose control over hospital environment and become dependent on the hospital personnel. This unknown, socially alienating situation not only makes women hesitant to seek hospital care, but also puts them to immense trouble on their arrival. People who can fearlessly walk in the darkness of the village become misplaced in the glowing light of the hospital due to structural design and the alien environment.

The urban-centric development of the hospital creates a distance from rural, poor women. In the Western world, urbanism influences the growth of hospitals with architectural, institutional and technical reorganisation to act as a curing machine (Foucault, 1980b, 1987). Proclivity to urbanism creates what Phillips (1990) terms a "health care hierarchy" (p. 106) in which facilities for better care are made available in urban areas. In this context, Paul (1983) points out that in

Bangladesh, the hierarchy of health facilities is associated with an urban-centric approach, with specialised care located at regional and district levels. As tertiary hospitals are associated with sophisticated treatment, prestige, and business, the dream of doctors is entwined with working in these hospitals. This also results in the development of hospitals in urban areas, with improved treatment facilities. In order to receive better care for birth complications, poor, rural families are compelled to seek cosmopolitan obstetric care by conceding to the harassment of spatial distance, which is reflected in multiple referrals through different health care hierarchies. However, these multiple referrals cause not only physical but also psychological exhaustion. A study in India documents the negative impact of multiple referrals on maternal mortality (Ganatra, Coyaji & Rao, 1998). Moreover, this geographically distant hospital also causes the expenditure of a fortune for rural families furthering their social distance.

Spatial distance and decision-making are the issues debated repeatedly in national and international discourses as disincentives to access hospital care (Sundari, 1992; Thaddeus & Maine, 1994). Yet, the reasons for low access to hospitals always seem to lie in the decision-making of families, not in the structural problems associated with urban-centric approach of health care hierarchies. Phillips (1990) argues that lack of political will and the power of elite classes favour urban bias in the organisation of hospitals. The political power of the urban rich is embedded in the urban-centric development of better service provision, not to mention that that doctors themselves are part of this powerful, elite society. Health care is hierarchised for the benefits of biomedical professionals as well as urban elites. Basic rights to obstetric care for birth complications are denied to rural, poor women due to the complicated politics of health care.

6.7 AUTHORITATIVE KNOWLEDGE OF BIOMEDICAL PROFESSIONALS

In cosmopolitan obstetrics, childbirth is legitimatised as a medical specialty (Oakley, 1979). According to Oakley (1980), giving birth in hospital means submitting oneself absolutely to medical authority. In this context, a metaphor taken from Mauriceau's (1668) *Maladies des Femmes Grosses*, provides an exemplar of the role of birthing women as opposed to the authority of doctors, "The pregnant woman is like a ship upon a stormy sea full of white caps and the good pilot who is in charge must guide her with prudence if he is to avoid shipwreck" (as cited in Taussig, 1937, as cited in Barker, 1998, p. 1067). It is this prudence of the pilot that is denoted as "authoritative knowledge" (Jordan, 1997, p. 56), which guides women while giving birth in hospital. With this background, my intent is to analyse what challenges are produced for rural women in confronting authoritative knowledge in hospital birth settings in Bangladesh.

Birth remains within the jurisdiction of biomedical professionals in hospitals (Oakley, 1979). Jordan's (1993) explication of authoritative knowledge in hierarchical settings of American hospitals establishes physician and medical staff as the dominant possessor of knowledge to the exclusion of birthing women. This authoritarian eminence of biomedical professionals is challenged by many scholars whose central concern is that women are subjected to the medical authority rendering them an impassive accomplice in their own birth experience (Davis-Floyd, 1990, 1992, 1994; Jordan, 1983, 1989, 1997; Kaufert & O'Neil, 1993; Kitzinger, 1982; Martin, 1989; Oakley, 1979, 1980; O'Neil & Kaufert, 1990; Rothman, 1982; Sargent, 1990). Social legitimation of authoritative knowledge is produced within the tremendous power imbalance that precludes women from taking active roles in the process of birth either by employing their knowledge or by expressing their decisions.

The dominance of biomedical professionals and the devaluation of birthing women are observed in medicalised birth events occurring in Bangladeshi hospitals. The authoritative knowledge of biomedical professionals developed on Baconian rationality of scientificity produces the "medical gaze" (Foucault, 1973, p. 137) that deeply infiltrates into rural women's body to know the invisible meaning, but not their clinical or personal realities (Nandy, 1995). In fact, rural women's bodies are "objectivised" into medicalised bodies by "dividing practices" (Foucault, 1982b, p. 208). As Foucault (1982b) describes, "The subject is either divided in himself or divided from others" (p. 208). Here, I can argue that technological, pharmacological and laboratory interventions take control over rural women to turn them into an "experimental" (Nandy, 1995, p. 154) bodies where biomedical professionals exercise manoeuvring, manipulation and mutilation in order to "govern" (Foucault, 1978, p.141) them. In the process, childbearing women are governed to deliver a baby, but their embodied knowledge is disqualified as "subjugated knowledge" (Foucault, 1980a, p. 81) and confined to the margins in erudite, medical domain. Jordan (1993) and Rothman (1982) observe women's positionality in hospital birth versus homebirth. In relation to hospital birth, Jordan comments, "She is not giving birth, she is delivered" (p. 165). On the other hand, Rothman states, "A woman at home is not delivered. She gives birth" (p.181). The arguments explicitly underpin the situation in Bangladesh where the dominant authoritative knowledge of biomedical professionals ascends over rural women's experiential knowledge making them marginal in their own birth experience.

Jordan (1997) explains authoritative knowledge as being "persuasive because it seems natural, reasonable and consensually constructed" (p. 59).[5] It means that in a birth setting, the knowledge that carries powerful authority is perceived by all the participants as natural and reasonable, since it is socially and consensually constructed (Jordan, 1993). In the context of Bangladesh, the establishment of doctors and nurses' knowledge as reasonable and natural is observed in rural women's submission to medical authority. It divulges their ostensible confidence in 'bookish' knowledge and medical competence in managing complications as opposed to experiential bodily knowledge that is seemingly redundant in hospital birth experience. In fact, the establishment of what is reasonable and natural is the result of the formation of "truth" (Foucault, 1987b, p.73) produced in the power struggles between women's subjugated knowledge and biomedical professionals' authoritative knowledge. According to the Foucauldian perspective, in modern, rational society, the truth of biomedical knowledge is developed from dominant scientific discourses, which are widely diffused, and established in societal demands (Cousins & Hussain, 1984). In this context, rural, poor women's docility to medical authority results from the truth produced by "bio-power" (Foucault, 1978, p. 140) of scientific, authoritative knowledge. Although it seems reasonable and natural, the construction of this authoritative knowledge on consensus raises suspicion. The appropriate term applicable in the Bangladeshi context is 'consensually accepted' rather than consensually constructed. Here, I may argue that the bio-power and truth of biomedical knowledge lead women to accept all the medical practices occurring in hospital consensually but in silence.

The authoritative knowledge of biomedical professionals is an established fact in the medical domain. In this context, Jordan (1997) asserts, "the power of authoritative knowledge is not that it is correct but that it counts" (p. 58). She continues to argue that it is the power of this medical dominance that makes this knowledge appear to be reasonable and neutral. Zola (1977) on the other hand, argues that the appeal of biomedical knowledge is its assumed moral neutrality, legitimising its relevance in curing diseases and resolving health problems. Oakley (1993) claims that the apparent moral neutrality of authoritative knowledge is seen as sufficient to dismiss women's knowledge and decisions as irresponsible. Their central concern is that authoritative knowledge is established with tacit, moral culpability to exercise rational, scientifically proven knowledge for women's benefit. Eventually, in the power struggles, rural women do not find any space to voice their problems or their wishes, as their knowledge is already discounted as ignorance in the medical domain. The authoritative knowledge under the cloak of competence (York, 1987) seems so reasonable, natural and morally neutral that increasing trends of caesarean sections, unnecessary episiotomy incisions, clinical iatrogenesis, and high, hospital, maternal death all remain unquestioned and are consensually accepted.

Rural women's absolute conformity to hospital obstetric practices is not always observed. Medical interventions have contributed to reducing mortality and morbidity in some childbirth complications (Jordan, 1983; Oakley, 1979). Complications of pregnancy and childbirth that cannot be managed by indigenous birth practices or indigenous medicine are managed in the domain of cosmopolitan obstetrics. Even then, rural women express non-conformity to prescribed medical practices. This non-conformity, in fact, is the "resistance" (Foucault, 1978, p. 95) of rural women to the authoritative knowledge of biomedical professionals, which is expressed in denial to seek hospital care, non-compliance with treatment, concealment of information and escape from the hospital. Bloor and Macintosh (1990) observed similar forms of resistance in therapeutic communities of Glasgow, where surveillance is carried out for health care. Avoidance of obstetric care and the prescribed medical rules are observed among birthing women across various cultures (Davis-Floyd, 1992; Martin, 1989; Whittaker, 2000). It is in this context, Foucault (1978) argues, that resistance is produced because bio-power cannot completely control matters due to the prevailing competing discourses. Rural women's versions and worldviews of birth offer competing discourses, which persuade them not to comply with and eventually to avoid hospital obstetric practices. This non-conformity is an expression of non-modern women's resistance to rational, scientific knowledge of modernity. In the following section, I shall discuss more about the resentment of rural women to cosmopolitan obstetrics in medical encounters.

6.8 THE TRIAD: DOCTOR, NURSE AND PATIENT

The role of doctors and nurses is as important in caring for patients as in curing diseases with the pattern of communication being influenced by their attitudes to patients. Oakley (1993), in this context, asserts that doctors present different faces to patients from different social class groups while their own social background influences communication with patients. A nurses' concern for social and psychological aspects of health means a better understanding of patients (Fisher, 1991). However, interpersonal relationships between nurses and doctors and within professions also have an effect on patient care. Here, I analyse how doctors and nurses behave with poor, rural women in medical encounters, why this pattern exists and how it causes resentment among women.

Interactions with patients are manifested in different forms in the everyday practices of doctors and nurses in Bangladeshi hospitals. In medical encounters, the communication of doctors with rural women is variable, but usually monologic, either silent or unsympathetic and abusive. Foucault (1973) argues that this silent pattern of communication is a reflection of the doctor's ways of knowing of the body. In fact, this biomedical knowledge delineates its exclusive focus to medical topics to the exclusion of women (Mishler, 1984). On the other hand, Lazaraus (1988) asserts that the knowledge of body and different expectations create their social distancing from patients. Their central observation is that the dominance of medical knowledge and the resultant social distancing affect the satisfying relationship between biomedical professionals and patients. This is certainly true of medical encounters in Bangladeshi hospitals. Few will dispute that work pressure and poor working environments contribute to this unsympathetic behaviour. Yet, the power of biomedical knowledge still remains predominant in medical encounters, as revealed in an Aberdeen hospital where the quality of interactions between health providers and patients remains unchanged even after increasing the consultation time (Porter, 1990). In this context, I may argue from a Foucauldian perspective that it is the power relations between biomedical professionals and rural, poor women that undermine the latter in medical encounters due to the disparity in knowledge and social distancing.

Careless attitudes to poor patients are predominantly observed in hospitals. The neglect to cultural values as observed by Jordan (1993) in Yucatan hospital birth practices is also manifested in Bangladeshi hospitals. Modesty, privacy and dignity are constantly infringed upon when women's vaginal and abdominal areas remain uncovered, and exacerbated by the presence of male doctors. The ways women's bodies are manipulated as if they were only vaginas. This rationalist knowledge of body-centric management sees rural women as machines not as human beings with emotional and psychological feelings (Martin, 1989; Oakley, 1993; Rothman, 1982). It is evident in biomedical professional's mere attention to freeing patients from diseases by overlooking their affording capacity to buy medicine (Kothari & Mehta, 1988). As patients are treated as malfunctioning biological organisms (Khuse, 1997), rural, poor women are, therefore, trapped in insensitive modern methods of treatment, where their cultural, personal and financial circumstances are overlooked.

The negligence of biomedical professionals is observed in providing treatment to patients. Clinical iatrogenesis inflicted by doctors and nurses regularly occurs in hospitals due to the unscientific practices, such as, use of non-sterilised instruments, not informing patients about the treatment process, and not attending patients in time. This carelessness falls into the category of medical malpractice (Annadale, 1996), but it remains unnoticed and unquestioned in hospitals. In this regard, Illich (1976) argues that societal dependence creates the unquestioned beliefs in the scientific practices of dominant, biomedical knowledge. His concern is that in the name of science and elitism, doctors are the strongest professional group in recent history whose errors seem acceptable. Like many developing countries, the negligence of biomedical professionals remains as a silent issue in Bangladesh due to the power of medical professions and the powerlessness of the patients.

Various reasons explain doctors' negligence in hospital wards. In the current context, patient's ignorance, doctor's work pressure and poor working environments are held responsible, which are also documented in research-based evidences in other countries (Annadale, 1996; Richman, 1987). Everyday practices of hospitals largely affect this behaviour (Foster & Anderson, 1978; Freidson, 1971; Konner, 1987; Richman, 1987) at the cost of poor woman's body. Doctor's negligence is greatly influenced by what Konner (1987) describes as the intentional pattern of socialisation of medical students in hospitals. Hahn and Gaines (1985) explicate the process of socialisation, which implicates medical schooling with doctors' learning "what is believed they should know" (p. 6). The scholars also assert that the informal process of socialisation has an effect on the continuation and modification of social interactions and rules within the socio-cultural milieu of medical institutions. Similarly, Richman (1987) buttresses the fact that the process of socialisation results from the socio-economic background of medical students, the impact of medical education and the immediate environment of hospital. Sometimes, biomedical professionals are not aware of their doings. In this context, Hudson-Rodd (1994) argues that medical and nursing students are developed with an understanding that, "Professional knowledge and good intentions would change the lives of the people for the better" (p.119). The process of socialisation in biomedical environment, therefore, has great influence in shaping doctor's attitudes to patients.

In Bangladeshi hospitals, neglectful attitudes of doctors to poor patients are observed in medical encounters. Junior doctors' association with unproblematic, elitist education and social living not only predestines their social distinctiveness, but also disallows them to cope with the crisis of a problematic world. In this problematic world, the dis-eased body embedded in indigence, illiteracy and rusticity is entrapped in a hospital, which is also stricken with poverty of resources and of morality. Here, I may argue that the behaviour and practices of doctors occur due to encountering a real problematic world, which is never taught in medical education and not learnt in economic affluence. It is concurrently exacerbated by their imitation of the manners exercised by senior doctors on poor patients. In addition, in a socially stratified society like Bangladesh, socialisation at home influences one's attitudes to the poor, which develop long before students' entrance to medical schools and are heightened by everyday practices of hospital milieu. All the issues work together to create neglectful attitudes of Bangladeshi doctors to rural, poor patients.

There is a difference between providing medical treatment and giving care to patients. Even though, the professional discourses of nursing claim that patients can only be cared for within the framework of their complex social and psychological lives (Fisher, 1991), providing medical treatment gives rise to a different situation. Porter (1990), in this context, argues that in hospitals, communications are based on medical dominance no matter who are the real caregivers. Her observation underscores the fact that midwives' behaviour to patients is similar to doctors in medical encounters. Despite the fact that most nurses in Bangladesh come from less affluent families, their behaviour in providing treatment to poor patients is influenced by the socialisation in hospitals, which over-rides the training they receive for patient care.

The role of nurses in Bangladeshi hospitals is challenged by their involvement in providing direct patient care. On the one hand, their continual negotiation with scarce supplies and hospital mismanagement, and, on the other hand, doctors' condescending attitudes demoralise them to the point where they revictimise and treat patients poorly. In fact, nurses are trapped in the social hierarchy of hospitals that arises from patriarchal order (Ehrenreich & English, 1973; Freidson, 1970; Porter, 1999; Turner, 1987). They are expected to take a great responsibility for patient care, but few have control over their work (Doyal, 1995). According to Freidson (1970), nurses are accorded with paraprofessional status that defers to the medical orders of doctors. In a similar vein, Khuse (1997) argues that doctors' higher status makes nurses dependent functionaries in patient care regardless of their professional and moral views. In fact, this situation is worsened when nurses are caught between multiple lines of authority in hospitals accountable both to doctors and bureaucratic administration (Schulz & Johnson, 1990). Under these circumstances, nurses in Bangladesh encounter problems in providing care to patients. Let me explain.

In hospitals, the nursing-in-charge constantly face challenges in managing wards and providing patient care because of the accountability to multiple authorities and the poor working environment. Despite their awareness of patients' needs and wants and the hospital situations, they are expected to follow doctors' commands and strict administrative rules. Even so, nurses take many decisions for patient care, particularly when doctors are not available or medicine orders are not refreshed. Negotiations with doctors and accountability for managerial tasks cause nurses' dissatisfaction. In this context, Johnstone (2002) argues that poor working environments and management structures cause stress and distress of nurses deteriorating their moral conscience and moral responsibility as care givers. The results are their unspoken disputes with doctors, senior colleagues and hospital administrators, and their persistent, visible disputes with patients and their families that eventually affect patient care.

Conflicts within professions also influence patient care. According to Schulz and Johnson (1990), a certain amount of conflict is beneficial to the organisations by creating changes and innovations, but on the other hand, the quality of patient care is adversely affected due to interpersonal conflicts. In Bangladeshi hospitals, conflicts among doctors and nurses result in poor service provision. Schulz and Johnson's (1990) arguments of conflicts are based on the unmet security or self-esteem in work, the disagreement with policies and practices, and the personal and emotional differences. In the given context, doctors' conflicts arise out of their frustrations and jealousy when they fail to achieve promotion, reputation, recognitions and business profit. On the other hand, the uncertainty of job expectations (Schulz & Johnson, 1990) creates silent conflicts between intern doctors and their immediate supervisors, which lead to increased work pressure, emotional stress and negligence to work among the formers. In a similar vein, student nurses in hospital wards negotiate with their immediate supervisors. Their outbursts against poor patients are occasionally evidenced due to emotional strain and work pressure. This situation, in fact, affects the working environment and eventually patient care.

Doctors and nurses are fostered in a modern, biomedical world where rationalist knowledge amalgamates with materialism, monetary gain and masculine traits. Yet, at the same time, medical professionals are exposed to age-old traditions of class systems and modern hierarchies of hospital organisation. Their values and judgement are shaped by their subjection to discursive practices (Foucault, 1978) occurring in the hospital environment and in everyday life. Then again, within the disciplining and struggling of modern institutions (Foucault, 1991a), the subjected, modern doctors/nurses encounter socially distant, rural, poor women possessing dissimilar worldviews. At the juncture of the modern and non-modern world, these power struggles result in muted or abusive interactions among modern health practitioners, and silent sufferings in non-modern, rural, poor women with their eventual resentment to cosmopolitan obstetric care.

6.9 FISCAL VIOLENCE

The tremendous costs of hospital services are a heartrending experience that rural, poor families face in seeking hospital obstetric care. The suddenness of expenditures put appaling demands on poor families, which Kothari and Mehta (1988) refer to as "fiscal violence" (p. 187). The combination of hospital costs and procedures on the one hand, and the circumstances of poverty, on the other, make rural women vulnerable to the fiscal violence of modern biomedical treatment. This issue I shall highlight to analyse why and how fiscal violence occurs to rural, poor women.

Despite the Bangladeshi Government's policy to provide free health care, the budgetary constraints of a developing country give rise to poorly resourced hospitals. This occurs not only because of a lack of resources, but also as a consequence of maldistribution of resources at different levels. Fewer resources are allocated and minimum level of services is rendered at the THC that covers more than eighty percent of the population. Within these parameters, poor distribution of resources influences discriminatory attitudes affecting the allocation to patient's treatment. About one percent of the annual hospital budget is allocated to patient treatment as opposed to other costs incurred in maintaining a mammoth hospital with its huge human resources (Anonymous, 2001c). Discrimination is intensified because of the need to manage the excessive number of patients in the context of the minimal resources allocated for sanctioned hospital beds. Scarcity is created because the budget is based on with the number of beds decided in the early sixties when the population size was less than one-third of the current size. Not only is the allocation of funds to health care very small, but also whatever is allotted cannot contribute to the improvement of health due to the demands of a growing population and rising health care expenditures.

The egalitarian approach of health care assumes provision of equal health services to the rich and poor, which collapses in inequitable service distribution. When the society is constrained by socio-economic inequalities and the budget is constrained by a maldistributive approach, the State's egalitarian approach in service allocation begets injustice to poor women. The State's policy is manipulated in the interests of upper class elites. Public hospital is the place where the poor seek care as a last resort. The rich usually attend private clinics. If the rich did use public hospitals, perhaps there would be better allocation of resources. However, the interests of the upper class are vested in their own profits. Their profit-making ventures combine with medical professionals' interests in making money from private clinics without regard for the health and development of the society as a whole. These factors give rise to a situation in which the poor get exploited not only due to social inequalities, but also due to futile policies of the State.

Lack of supplies in hospitals put doctors in an advantageous position to prescribe drugs from a particular pharmaceutical company. In Bangladesh, 62 percent of total medical expenditures are associated with drug expenses (Bangladesh Bureau of Statistics, 1999). In contrast, drugs account for about 11 percent of the National Health Service (NHS) spending in Britain (Doyal, 1979). A research conducted in Bangladesh demonstrates that 55 percent of expenditures on caesarean sections are attributed to drugs only (Nahar & Costello, 1998). Prescribing medicine from pharmaceutical companies is not only linked to receiving bribes from them, but also to the absolute, unquestioning belief of doctors in their documented reports (Chowdhury, 1996). The practice of drug prescription was commonly observed in the hospitals during my fieldwork. The enormous expenditures on drugs attract multinational pharmaceutical companies to invest in developing countries (Doyal, 1979). Doctors in Bangladeshi hospitals are trapped in the profit-making ventures of multinational pharmaceutical companies to the detriment of poor patients. Fiscal violence, thus, occurs due to the cost explosion of modern treatment attributing to high-tech diagnostic and treatment facilities and pharmaceutical products (Doyal, 1979; Phillips & Verhasselt, 1994). Eventually, the poor become poorer by getting caught in the web of politics of biomedical and pharmaceutical practices.

Under-resources in hospitals create space for paying unofficial fees, stealing hospital supplies and misusing services, which can be called "dirty work" (p. 161) at the back stage (Turner, 1987) or corruption (Nye, 1970, as cited in Rose-Ackerman, 1978). Paying unofficial fees is evident in many hospitals across Bangladesh and India (Chowdhury, Mahbub & Chowdhury, 2002; Jeffery, Jeffery & Lyon, 1989; Killingsworth, et al., 1999; Leppard, 2000). Although some argue that poorly paid staff are involved in it, in these hospitals doctors and nurses are also involved. The continuation of this process in hospitals is buttressed by Wilsford's (1991) argument about the existence of different interest groups who possess both private and public interests. Rose-Ackerman (1999) argues that it is the self-interest or greed that provokes individuals or groups to become involved in corruption. The poor, salaried staff are a vulnerable group who are easily bribed, but corrupt practices also serve the interests of high-level officials (Rose-Ackerman, 1978). In Bangladeshi hospitals, the persistence of corruption among the poorly paid staff not only serves their personal interests, but also benefits particular interest groups who are not directly involved. However, Kohli (1975) argues that middle and lower level staff imitate the ways of their seniors, as the senior staff initiate to resort to corrupt practices. In Bangladesh, the silence of hospital administration is due to their political and personal interests. This analysis is supported by Chowdhury's (1996) detailed documentation of the politics of drugs in Bangladesh where different officials including doctors partake in corrupt practices of money-making. Corruption is not always directly related to earning cash, fulfilment of political interests is also executed by being involved in it (Dutt, 1975). It can, therefore, be argued that it is the interests of different groups that ignore the unofficial earning of doctors and nurses for their professional solidarity and political interests. In the process, a structure is created in which all the corruptive practices occurring in hospitals become acceptable. Ahmed (2001), in this context claims, "Corruption, therefore, is not merely a financial transaction or some bending of rules but the very reproduction of the structure that goes on to make such a transaction or bending of rules possible" (p. 21). Entrapped within this structure, the hospitals are crippled with poor service quality that eventually causes poor, rural women to bear the burdens of financial, physical and psychological sufferings while receiving obstetric care.

Modern, biomedical treatment is economically and socially distant from the poor. The majority in Bangladesh do not have the capacity to bear the expenditures due to their impoverished state. Maldistribution of resources, lack of supplies, corruption, and urban-centric development of hospitals all combine to cause huge costs in modern obstetric treatment. The cost of caesarean section is four to five times the monthly income of 76 percent of households that earn less than Tk. 5000 per month (Bangladesh Bureau of Statistics, 1999). This high cost is not unique to Bangladesh as the costs of caesarean sections in India exceed many families' monthly income by four times (Jeffery, Jeffery & Lyon, 1989). In a similar vein, the costs incurred in normal birth in Medical College Hospital are close to the monthly income of some families. Rural, poor women are accustomed to birth experience in their own domain with the support of family members and other women. On occasion, they die or suffer. But, when they seek care from hospitals, the sudden, immense expenditures trap them with fiscal violence. Even if their lives are saved, women turn into inanimate living beings handicapped with poverty and hunger. Arguing with the exorbitant expenditures of modern treatment and its effectiveness, Kothari and Mehta (1988) assert, "it is the family that has to be buried" (p, 175) for expending their last penny in India. In USA, where there is no universal public health care system, every fifth case of personal bankruptcy occurs as people are forced to pay the large medical bills (Kothari & Mehta, 1988). These hefty expenses, especially for caesarean sections and other major operations, result in acute crisis in poor families leading to further starvation and absolute poverty. The national and global efforts to improve maternal health have little meaning to poor women whose families become morbid victims of modern, biomedical treatment. This situation results in fiscal violence for families already incapacitated by hunger and poverty exacerbated by modernity and capitalism in a post-colonial State like Bangladesh. In the next section, I shall discuss how the post-colonial modern State contributes to more sufferings of rural, poor women.

6.10 WOMEN, STATE AND OBSTETRIC CARE

Childbirth is not a disease, but a normal event. Neither hospitalisation nor antenatal care reduces the number of maternal deaths (Tew, 1990). Even so, the colonised mentality of the State, enchanted with the scientific rationality of modern medicine patronises its development and seeks to medicalise birth experiences. It is the State that brings modernity into the understanding of health care and that utilises its resources to transform the health care in its own image. Indeed, in the context of South Asia, including Bangladesh, colonial legacy and neo-colonial invasion strengthen the position of biomedicine as a representation of modernity. It is against this background that I shall analyse how the childbirth experiences of rural women are addressed in modern State of Bangladesh.

The medical profession is established in the context of the social, economic and political forces developed in the modern State. In discussing the power of the modern State, Chatterjee (1993) argues, from the Foucauldian perspective, that it is the advance of a 'modern' regime of power that facilitates and produces more power of the colonial legacy in postcolonial India. His argument is that the postcolonial State shaped and patterned by the precise rules and techniques left by the colonisers are the power of modernity manipulated in the modern State. It is this power of the modern State that influences modern obstetric practices in postcolonial Bangladesh. That espousal of the modern State renders the medical profession a powerful, professional group not only by delegating full authority to possess knowledge of the body and to control the health of the population, but also by creating space for medical education and practices (Foucault, 1980b). In fact, this concentrated, elitist knowledge makes the profession dominant because of its overriding monopoly that precludes other forms of knowledge (Illich, 1977). At the same time, modern capitalism adds monetary value to the medical profession conferring on it a higher societal status. As a result, in Bangladesh, the policy and planning concerning childbirth issues are accorded with the ideas of medical profession that facilities modern, obstetric practices in hospitals and creates a speciality no matter how useful it is for childbearing women. The recent policy of Safe Motherhood Initiatives supported by WHO is geared to increase skilled, birth attendance in which people with proficient midwifery skills such as doctors, nurses and midwives are accountable to manage normal deliveries and refer complications (World Health Organisation, 1999). This influences the State to initiate the training of new generations of literate midwives who will soon be introduced into the community (Ministry of Health and Family Welfare, 1998a). The WHO approach, in fact, supports modern biomedicine. It is in this context, I can argue that the State and the WHO influenced by modernity patronise cosmopolitan obstetrics, and attempt to eliminate the already marginalised *dainis* condemned as dirty, ignorant and failed by facilitating this modern approach which Wagner (1995) terms as "global witch-hunt" (p. 1020). The WHO has lost its philosophy developed on primary health care when it was born in 1946 and reaffirmed by the Alma Ata declaration in 1978.

The establishment and continuation of modern obstetrics result from the State's intervention in serving the interests of different groups. In developed societies, historical evidence suggests that the professional, business and male-dominated interests of medical professions jeopardise traditional midwifery with the support of the State (Ehrenreich & English, 1973). In this context, Doyal (1979) argues that the medical profession in postcolonial countries is established and maintained because upper class elites retain this colonial legacy as a mark of prestige. This prestige is nothing but 'subjectivity' to modern biomedical knowledge that exercises power on this particular class to establish its legitimacy as well as produces the pride of being 'modern'. Yet, this issue of being modern is not only located in the upper class, but it is also transmitted to the middle class because the latter imitates the former (Navarro, 1981). On the other hand, Oakley (1984) argues that medical hegemony over patient's lives becomes substantial, as dependency on medical professions increases. In fact, in postcolonial Bangladesh, the institution and continuation of modern obstetrics are due to societal dependence (Illich, 1976) of the ruling upper class enhanced by the patronising attitudes of the State. It is in this context, I can argue from Foucauldian perspectives, that the State subjected to the discourses of modernity and modern biomedical knowledge serves the interests of upper class elites who are subjected to the same knowledge to establish and continue modern obstetrics in Bangladesh.

The State has given full autonomy to medical professions by providing opportunities for their practice (Doyal, 1979). While the State places control over social and economic organisation of medical work, it "leaves the profession control over technological side" (Oakley, 1984, p.256). In Bangladesh, there is no control or supervision of medical practices by the State. Illich's (1977) argument about the role of medical professions in modern State seems appropriate. In this context, he claims, "They turn the modern State into a holding corporation of enterprises which facilitates the operation of their self-certified competencies" (p.16). This control is reflected in hospitals of Bangladesh where the monopoly of the medical professionals is so dominant that their technological, economic and social activities are never questioned or scrutinised by the State. It is the power of biomedical knowledge that makes all the events natural and acceptable by objectifying the State as well as the public to be subjected to it. This continuation of the process eventually affects the poor, rural women whose visions and versions are already silenced in power struggles with the authoritative knowledge of biomedical professionals.

The most important issue addressed in health policy and planning with regard to childbirth is the reduction of maternal mortality and morbidity. Here, we can observe that the State policy is geared towards modern obstetric care allocating the total budgetary resources by organising different programmes in health care hierarchies. Yet, the resources used for obstetric care are not at all adequate for the women for whom it is intended. In Bangladesh, more than 90 percent of births occur at home. Of the total estimated annual births, only 5.33 percent take place at government health facilities and 2.93 percent at private clinics when a minimum of 15 percent are expected to happen in hospitals (Khan, Kanam, Nahar, Nasrin, & Rahman, 2000). When the

State cannot afford to provide adequate obstetric services to five percent of cases, it would be a dreadful situation, if the predicted 15 percent complications of births seek public hospital obstetric care. The under resourcing of hospitals occurs not just because of the "lack of resources" in the country "but who has control over these resources" (Navarro, 2000, p. 673). This is reflected in the maldistribution of resources at a national level where the defence budget (13%) is about three times of the health budget (5%) (Ministry of Finance, 2002). In this context, Navarro (1981, 2000) argues that this situation occurs to meet the self-interests of lumpen-bourgeois who themselves participate in maintaining the power of the State. Moreover, maldistribution in health care hierarchies arises from facilitating the urban-centric, medical practices that benefit the upper class societies as well as medical professions (Phillips, 1990). Poor resources in annual hospital budget for patient care give rise to poor, quality, hospital services with a lack of supplies and facilities that not only impede patient care, but also result in an unclean hospital environment encouraging infections and cross-infections. Even if women survive, their impoverished bodies are worsened by fiscal violence and incapacitated by hospital morbidities.

Childbirth is medicalised, turned into a commodity in modern, capitalist society. It is the State that facilitates modern, obstetric practices because the whole medical system has become a business enterprise. In this business enterprise, medical professions, pharmaceutical companies, technological factories, laboratories, hospitals and clinics all are involved (Sanders & Carver, 1985). These elites monopolise this business throughout the world and at the same time, facilitate funding to the international NGOs as well as the projects in the developing countries. The globalised, market economy enhances the flourishing of medical professions and modern obstetrics for their own benefits, and the State, in this context, plays an intermediary role to facilitate the process (Doyal, 1979, 1995). Thus, like many developing countries, whatever resources are allocated for the improvement of maternal health in Bangladesh used to serve the interests of capitalist, market economy in which cosmopolitan obstetric practices are intertwined, but indigenous birth practices are not.

The focus on medical professions and under-resourced, hospital structures diverts attention from the underlying causes of maternal mortality and morbidity. While the causes of maternal mortality and morbidity are debated, the significance of socio-economic contexts is ignored with little effort undertaken to address the issues in Bangladesh. In developed countries, maternal mortality is reduced not simply due to better access to obstetric care, but to better education, better nutrition, improvements in housing and working conditions, and wider availability of effective, birth control (Doyal, 1995; McKeown, 1989). In Bangladesh, poor women are deprived of the social facilities that enhance their socio-economic conditions. Moreover, the impoverishment of the postcolonial State still carries the trait of exploitation from the colonial period due to the drain of wealth, the destruction of productive systems and the creation of a backward economy (Chatterjee, 1993). Later, in the postcolonial period, as experienced by all developing countries, this State becomes the victim of the neo-colonial invasion of modern, capitalist, market economy. It is the modern State, regardless of its economic status, facilitates the upper class economy eventually giving rise to increasing social inequalities (Navarro & Shi, 2001). It is reflected in the current situation of Bangladesh where the level of consumption expenditure inequality increases from 30.7 to 36.8 percent in urban areas and from 24.3 to 27.1 percent in rural areas (Ministry of Finance, 2002). When the poor become poorer, there is less scope for improving maternal health only by reorganising cosmopolitan obstetric care, which is equally inefficient in improving maternal health.

Bangladesh is a modern State. It is the power of modernity that shapes ideas and practices of the State influencing the health policy and planning. The *techne* of the State denoted as "bio-power" (Foucault, 1978), is intended to improve maternal health, but, the power struggles of different discursive practices occurring in the social, economic and political contexts give rise to a situation where poor, rural women agonise. Foucault (1991b), in fact, condemns the present situation of modernity as the "governmentalisation of the State" (p. 103), where the problems of governmentality and the techniques of government turn into political issues and the space for political struggles. He argues that the tactics of governmentality define and redefine the survival and limits of the State, which are internal and external to the State. It is in this context, I can argue from the Foucauldian perspective, that the health policy and planning for the reduction of maternal mortality and morbidity become the space for political struggles and contestations of different groups, individuals and institutions due to the problems of governmentality occurring within and outside the control of the State. Within power struggles, this modern State acknowledges and strengthens modern, obstetric practices while marginalises indigenous birth practices. This eventually results in a situation where the State's approaches to reducing maternal mortality and morbidity turn into a charade for rural, poor women for whom it is intended.

6.11 SUMMARY AND CONCLUSION

The intent of the research is to explore why and in what ways rural, poor women adhere to indigenous birth practices and resist cosmopolitan obstetric care. This analysis explicates childbirth experiences in the contexts of culture, gender, socio-economy, political economy and history. Understanding of birth, women's silence, the mind/body unification and embodied knowledge are produced in a socio-cultural context that persuades women to adhere to indigenous birth practices. Yet, the unfixity of birth meaning makes women undecided about seeking medical care in the event of a birth crisis. At times, this leads to fatal consequences. This situation is worsened by their silence causing more suffering in birth experiences. On the other hand, the mind/body unification and the embodied experience of birth provide women with immense knowledge to actively engage in birth events. Even then, women suffer from uncertain consequences of birth, which, in fact, lead them to search for different options of care.

When rural women seek refuge in cosmopolitan obstetric care, particularly during times of birth complications, their knowledge is precluded by the dominant, authoritative knowledge of modern obstetrics. In facing modern, birthing care, they become inactive accomplices in their own birth experiences and remain silent with further physical and psychological sufferings.

Indigenous knowledge of birth is communal knowledge, in which each woman participates and mutually exchanges knowledge. Although, birthing women play a significant role in the birth event, *dainis* with indigenous skills provide them with physical, emotional and psychological supports. This supportive relationship between women and *dainis* is not based on a hierarchy of knowledge or materialistic gain. In contrast, the interpersonal relationship among women, doctors and nurses is predicated on monopolistic, medical knowledge and professional hierarchies exacerbated by materialistic values. Despite the supportive relationship existing between *dainis* and women, indigenous knowledge of birth is challenged by cosmopolitan obstetric practices supported by the modern State. Not only is the knowledge of *dainis* marginalised, but they themselves also become apprehensive of their role and suffer from an identity crisis and confidence on the brink of modernity. On the contrary, the authoritative knowledge of cosmopolitan obstetrics situates itself at the zenith of modernity with medical dominance.

Authoritative, biomedical knowledge is monopolistic. It denies space for the existence of other forms of knowledge. It requires mammoth hospital buildings and urban proclivity for the flourishing of biomedical professions. This grandness does not mean that the quality of services is good. Maldistribution of resources and corrupt practices give rise to poor quality services in Bangladeshi hospitals. As a result, poor women, already incapacitated by poverty, are trapped in further poverty caused by fiscal violence incurred in hospital obstetric treatment.

The State is modern. It patronises medical professions because its philosophy coincides with that of modern biomedicine, which is based on scientific rationalism, technology, capitalism and patriarchy. Despite the roots of maternal mortality and morbidity being embedded in socio-economic causes, the health policy and planning geared to a medical model of health facilitates the medicalisation of childbirth.

Rural women, nurtured in indigenous ways of living seek assistance from indigenous birthing care because their visions and versions are similar. These women are distant from cosmopolitan obstetrics because the latter is tied up with diametrically opposed, knowledge of birth, elitism and monetary values. Seeking cosmopolitan obstetric care, therefore, makes rural, poor women the victims of physical, psychological, fiscal and political violence.

What to do? A study of this nature seeks to describe the world, but is this enough? In the next, and final, chapter, not only is the research question answered but also directions for future research and praxis are made that support women in giving birth safely. As Karl Marx once said, the point is not just to understand the world, the point is to change it.

Notes

[1] The women-to-women support gives rise to self-help group where women discuss and resolve their own health problems.

[2] Chatterjee (1993) continues his discussion with home and world, which correspond with the spiritual aspect of traditional India and the material

aspect of the Western world. The colonised men in India incorporate them into the materialistic world of Western patriarchal dominance for their material development, but never admit it in their spiritual world. They relocate their spiritual aspect inside the home where women are particularly represented. Women who represent home remain in traditional patriarchal dominance maintain feminine qualities and men exposed to the world accept the material aspect of Western patriarchy based on science, technology, rationalism and capitalism. This gives an understanding of social roles by gender to correspond with the separation of the social space into *ghar* (home) and *bahir* (world).

3 It is note worthy that paying cash for physical service is also not practiced even for male healers and health practitioners in villages. Payment is made only for material services, such as selling medicine or giving amulets. Besides, for spiritual healing, payment is made on client's satisfaction.

4 It was intended to train one TBA for each of 68,000 villages or one for 1500 population. According to Akhter, Rahman, Mannan, Elahi, & Khan (1995), 42,185 TBAs were trained by 1994.

5 This definition is constructed considering both community and hospital practices, where she continues to argue that in community practices, people are actively and confidently engaged in knowledge production, but on the other hand, in hospital their knowledge is excluded.

Chapter 7

Epilogue and the Future

When I finished my fieldwork, I was asked by an eminent person in Bangladesh what would be drawn from this research. I kept silent for a while looking outside, through the window. Suddenly, I visualised the events in *Apurbabari*, the THC and the Medical College Hospital like snapshots one after another, and listened to the multiple voices, but, most of all, those of the women. At that juncture, I did not know what I could infer from narrowing down all the experiences that had a much broader focus. After meticulously considering my research experience, I contemplate the emergence of new hopes, aspirations and desires combined with compassion for the rural, poor women, for whom the research is intended. In the conclusion, I review research findings, explore the significance of these findings, suggest future research directions and offer central areas for changes in childbirth practices of Bangladesh.

I began the research with the aim of exploring why and in what ways rural, poor women in Bangladesh adhere to indigenous birth practices and, concurrently, resist cosmopolitan obstetrics. I employed ethnographic methods, particularly in-depth interviews and participant observations to gather information in one village, the adjacent THC and the Medical College Hospital. I have argued that in order to understand the complexities of childbirth, a multidimensional framework encompassing culture, gender, socio-economic, political economy and historical perspectives must be considered. Situating childbirth in this framework, I have analysed indigenous birth practices and cosmopolitan obstetrics where the construction of birth is defined and redefined in discursive practices that shape rural, poor women's use of birthing care. The overall aim of the study is to improve childbirth practices in Bangladesh by recognising women's active roles in birth; acknowledging indigenous knowledge; highlighting social, cultural, economic and political influences that affect women's health and health care during birth experiences; integrating indigenous birthing care with cosmopolitan obstetrics in a manner that is sensitive to women's needs; and improving the organisation of the existing health care system.

The findings of the study identify key issues related to birth practices. In *Apurbabari*, women understand the birth process as *thikmoton* (usual) or *kolbekol* (difficult). As birth is naturally expected to happen, it normally takes place at home. Difficult births are attempted at home and if this trial fails and complications eventuate, birthing women are taken to hospital. This occurs due to plural, unfixed understandings of birth that are influenced by everyday practices in the village. These understandings of birth make them undecided about seeking appropriate care in a birth crisis, and, at times, lead to fatal consequences of mother and child.

Maintaining silence during pregnancy, and specifically during birth, is identified as an important issue related to their notions of *sharam*, which is meant to sustain privacy. Yet, this silence causes more sufferings in birth experiences, especially when there are problems. In their birth experience women sustain *moner shahosh* (mental strength) and *shoriler shakti* (physical strength) and focus on comprehending the bodily mechanisms. The mind/body unification and the embodied experience of birth provide women with immense knowledge to actively engage in their own birth events, but with uncertain consequences. In indigenous birth, the uncertainty in birth consequences eventually leads them to search for different options of care.

When seeking refuge in cosmopolitan obstetric care, particularly for birth complications, rural, poor women and their families face continual predicaments from admission to discharge, especially in the Medical College Hospital. They are forced to search hither and thither for assistance in an unfamiliar environment, face doctors' condescending attitudes and nurses' rude behaviour, and bear huge expenditures in treatment. Moreover, the actual experience of hospital birth produces resentful feelings among rural, poor women that become part of village, cultural expectations about hospital birth.

The experiences of hospital birth are totally different from the home birth experiences. Women's knowledge is precluded by the dominant, authoritative knowledge of modern obstetrics rendering them inactive and unimportant accomplices in their own birth experiences. A few doctors and nurses demonstrate their caring concern for the poor patients. Nevertheless, the preponderance of neglectful attitudes and misconduct humiliate birthing women. This interpersonal relationship between women and biomedical professionals may be explained in a number of ways: monopolised, biomedical knowledge, the enculturation of doctors into their professional hierarchical roles, and the materialistic values of the professionals in hospitals. Moreover, scarce resources and corrupt practices including influences of pharmaceutical companies on doctors put poor families under tremendous pressure to bear the huge expenditures incurred in hospital treatment. All these issues work together to give rise to poor, service quality in hospitals. Under these circumstances, rural, poor women suffer silently with resentment in face of modern, birthing care.

The findings also suggest that indigenous knowledge of birth is communal knowledge, which women mutually exchange. The role of each woman in providing physical and emotional support becomes visible through sharing of knowledge and experiences. In the context of this support, birthing women play a significant, active role in their own birth event. Also crucial is the participation of *dainis*, who not only apply indigenous skills in facilitating the birthing process, but also share their supportive role. The trust and dependence of women on *daini's* skills and supports and the horizontal, non-hierarchical relationship among women make the former indulge in the latter while experiencing birth.

The study concludes that childbirth is constructed in discursive practices occurring in the social world, which influence rural, poor women's use of birthing care. Understanding of birth, women's silence, *sharam* and privacy, mind/body unification, embodied knowledge, and active participation in birth, and trust and dependence on *dainis'* skills persuade women to adhere to indigenous birth practices. On the other hand, the authoritative knowledge of biomedical professionals, the medicalised experience of birth, the interpersonal relationships, hospital costs, and varied experiences in an alien hospital environment cause women to resist use of cosmopolitan obstetrics and strengthen their adherence to indigenous birth practices.

7.1 THIS RESEARCH AND THE SIGNIFICATION

The significance of the research results lies in the emerging depiction of childbirth practices in Bangladesh. Through careful documentation of ethnographic details of two contemporary birthing practices and their critical analysis within a multidimensional framework, I have demonstrated that the women's voice primarily unravels their experiences of birth practices at home and in hospitals. The diversity of indigenous knowledge is exemplified by the experiences of *dainis*. On the other, the participation of doctors, nurses and other hospital staff contributes to illuminate many practices occurring in hospitals. More importantly, my observational experiences reinforce multi-voiced, homogenous and heterogenous experiences explaining the context of birth practices at home and in hospitals.

The use of a Foucauldian perspective has revealed the power of knowledge created in discursive practices that objectify rural women, biomedical professionals and even the State. The multiple, power structures maintaining discipline on the woman's body allow for control of the woman's natural processes of birth by the biomedical professionals. The critical issues raised in the study should be considered before initiating further research and introducing programmes related to childbirth in Bangladesh.

One of the important findings in this study is the paradox existing between the non-modern and modern worlds of birth practices. The paradox is that rural, poor women constantly feel threatened and disgraced in facing the modern world and indigenous knowledge of birth is marginalised on the brink of modernity. I have argued that the distinctiveness of the study lies in the recognition of indigenous knowledge of birth as a communal knowledge and acknowledges women's active roles in their birth event. The study reveals the hidden, self-help approach existing in indigenous birth practices through which women share their experiences, enrich their bodily knowledge and participate in birth. Engaging women's experiential and embodied knowledge is important, and needs to be stressed, not only in addressing childbirth issues, but also in recognising other health-related problems. The study also brings to light indigenous skills of *dainis*, which exist as deprofessionalised care without monetary gain within the domain of home.

The results of this study should not be taken as romanticising indigenous knowledge. Not all indigenous practices are acceptable such as, using unwashed hands in touching the birth canal. More importantly, indigenous practices are not adequate for managing complicated births. In fact, some cultural understandings of birth impede women's access to appropriate care. The outcome can mean fatal consequences for mother and baby.

Access to appropriate care during birth complications is a vital issue. The outcomes of this study have shown that cosmopolitan obstetrics, as currently practiced in Bangladesh, are neither appropriate nor adequate. This study reveals the details of obstetric practices in hospitals, which include: medicalised, birth experience; authoritative, biomedical knowledge; intimidating, interpersonal relationship between biomedical professionals and rural, poor women; corrupt practices; the manipulative role of pharmaceuticals; enormous, treatment costs; and alien environment. At the same time, this supposedly scientific method of obstetric care gives rise to unscientific practices in local, hospital environments. The research has recognised the importance of deprofessionalising biomedical professions and the concerted commitment of doctors, nurses, different individuals and groups to improve hospital practices.

I have sought to reveal how modernity, capitalism, rationality and patriarchy shape birth practices in hospitals to create widely divergent birth experiences with physical, psychological and fiscal sufferings for non-modern women who resist access to modern, obstetric care. Another significant feature of the research is that the role of the State becomes visible in supporting modern cosmopolitan obstetrics and eliminating indigenous birth practices. The policy formulation, programme implementation and resource allocation of the State reveal its endorsement of the development and continuation of modern birth practices.

But where is the balance? For example, I have argued that Safe Motherhood Initiatives, rather than working within the framework of socio-economic and cultural context of women's lives, are in fact, being used as medical tools to bring changes in birth practices that accord with cosmopolitan obstetrics. This completely ignores the roots of maternal death and disease and also marginalises indigenous birth practices. It is clearly evident in this research that birth practices, from micro to macro levels, are shaped and patterned by the power struggles occurring in discursive practices that influence rural, poor women's adherence to indigenous birth practices and resistance to cosmopolitan obstetrics.

7.2 FUTURE RESEARCH SKETCH

This study has revealed and broadened the scope for further research on childbirth practices. The significance of future research on indigenous birth practices is that it will explore and enrich knowledge and strengthen the space for its development and sustainability in the face of modernity. The diversity of indigenous knowledge of birth is highlighted in the study, yet further research is required to exemplify and explicate comprehensively specific themes that arose in the study. For example, genealogical studies will be important to explore the embodied experience of birth as well as the indigenous skills of *dainis* in order to identify the profundity of the existing resources of knowledge. Moreover, the need for an intense exploration of birth is crucial, particularly the ethnographic details of the management of birth complications because rural women face persistent problems in making decisions about appropriate care. The issue of *sharam* is an area of interest for further research in relation to women and body. Cultural knowledge of birth practices have yet to be explored to illuminate the plurality of understandings, particularly, the concept of death, food taboos, evil spirits and pollution. Future research should incorporate the cross-country and cross-cultural research to compare and contrast the strengths and weakness of indigenous birth practices. Inter-religion comparison is also important to document the diverse knowledge and practices of birth. This will provide a repository of knowledge that may contribute to enriching indigenous birth practices. More importantly, the continuity of research is encouraged in this field to improve indigenous birth skills.

Research in cosmopolitan obstetrics is equally essential to improve medical, obstetric practices. The need for understanding the birth experiences of caesarean section patients in Bangladesh is paramount. This study indicates that doctors' authoritarian attitudes need to be explored from their own perspectives. Genealogical studies in this field may explicate changes over time in doctor's attitudes. It is also crucial to explore comprehensively their understandings of birth and the issues of medicalisation and their knowledge about indigenous birth practices. Participatory, action research should be conducted to raise the awareness of doctors and to abolish hierarchical structures of knowledge. Nursing professions also face challenges in hospitals. In this regard, individual in-depth studies in this profession may inform us about nurses' changing attitudes to and practices in patient care.

The qualitative nature of the present study has demonstrated the continuing importance of comprehensive research into the causes of maternal morbidity and mortality in hospitals. Identical community based studies are required to elucidate maternal morbidities and mortalities. On the other hand, research on the increasing trends of caesarean sections is considered essential to question the worth and significance of this intervention. Such studies challenge the root causes of hospital deaths and morbidities.

There is, of course, an essential gender element needed in all future research that will include not only an exploration of birthing women but also of their caregivers. There is a need, for example, to investigate special *ayahs'* silent sufferings as women in hospitals. Such research may need to focus on issues of sexual harassment. Female obstetricians' status among medical professionals is another area required to be studied.

Research on medical bureaucracies is worth pursuing in order to understand the management and administration problems. Corrupt practices in hospitals are a regular phenomenon. These issues require investigation because it not only causes fiscal violence among poor patients seeking hospital care, but also raises the question of moral decay at societal level.

In summary, future directions for research on childbirth issues need to recognise the importance of conducting ethnographic and epidemiological studies over a period of time and in different locations as being essential to fully comprehend childbirth practices. Our present understanding of birth practices can only be strengthened by cross-cultural research to identify the strengths and rectify the weaknesses, which eventually will improve birthing experiences for all women.

7.3 WHAT CHANGES CAN BE MADE IN FUTURE BIRTH

Women's needs and expectations during childbirth can be addressed by making changes or innovations in both indigenous birth and cosmopolitan obstetric practices. In the light of earlier discussion and arguments, I propose some recommendations at local as well as at broader levels with the aim of improving childbirth practices in Bangladesh that may lead to better maternal health. In order to improve maternal health, mere changes in health care do not sufficiently address this issue. In this context, Hudson-Rodd (1994) suggests that in achieving health, issues of equity, relations of power and knowledge, and public and professional participation are important. The principles of the recommendations are based on: acknowledging women's indigenous knowledge; integrating indigenous birthing care and cosmopolitan obstetrics to create sensitive health care for women; improving the organisation of the existing health care system; and creating space to improve maternal health. The approaches applied to make innovations are comparable to strategies proposed in the Ottawa Charter for Health Promotion (World Health Organisation, 1986). It includes: building healthy public policy; creating supportive environments; strengthening community action; developing personal skills; and reorienting health services. In consideration of the findings of my research, I propose to accentuate the following areas to create a supportive context of childbirth.

Women's Role in Birth

Empowering women strengthens their role in childbirth. Women in indigenous birth are already empowered. The issue of empowering women's role in birth brings into light: active engagement in birth; understandings of birth; silence in birth; and indigenous skills. To reinforce indigenous knowledge of birth, these issues can be addressed through self-help approach. The underlying principles of this self-help approach are based on developing capacity and confidence in self-care through sharing knowledge and experiences (Doyal, 1995). As rural women are seen to acquire knowledge and confidence through experiences and circumstances, the self-help approach will be useful to acknowledge and strengthen women's power of giving birth. These interactions addressing the significance of mind/body unification and embodied knowledge not only strengthen women's knowledge, but also create a supportive group before birth takes place. On the other hand, the role of indigenous, patriarchal dominance in women's silence at home birth is a crucial issue needing thorough discussion in groups to make women aware of health and social problems. In similar vein, the discussion on the importance of identifying and referring difficult birth to appropriate medical care in time will be encouraged. However, as birth is considered as a private matter, small groups within the family sphere, or similar age group circles, will facilitate participatory and effective discussions. The self-help approach will clarify many issues for women and augment their knowledge that eventually reinforces their role in birth.

Empowering women's role in birth draws attention to improving indigenous skills. Indigenous birth is communal knowledge shared by all women participating in the event. Although *dainis* possess immense skills of birth, they are not sufficient to manage normal birth. In this context, the integration of indigenous birth and cosmopolitan obstetrics is seen as relevant in which biomedical knowledge on asepsis and birth complications should be incorporated into indigenous birth practices in a locally understandable manner. Issues of improving indigenous skills can be discussed in self-help group discussion at home. However, as *dainis* learn from experiences and circumstances, this knowledge cannot be transmitted through a simple didactic approach. Rather, learning by doing (Jordan, 1983), otherwise known as action learning, may facilitate the development of *dainis'* skills.

Community Support for Birth

In the quest for improving and strengthening birth practices, a crucial task is to organise a structure in the community that sustains these activities. Such community-based organisation should deploy the services and skills of NGOs or women's organisations by strengthening community support to maternal health. These processes built up by the members of the community, essentially aim to empower women. However, they cannot be operated in terms of target achieving approach that is associated with contemporary funding opportunities.

In order to strengthen indigenous birth practices, the associated community organisations will need to preserve indigenous knowledge in archives and remain conscious about not medicalising birth process and not professionalising existing traditions of birth practices. Knowledge is power, so an advocacy organisation must be equipped with full information related to women's health. It will empower women in the community by strengthening their knowledge of birth and other health-related matters, including socio-economic and cultural issues. This will assist women to seek appropriate health care and to search for resolution of social and economic problems.

Seeking care from hospital is constrained by many issues that are not related to indigenous knowledge. The transfer to hospital for birth complications could be hastened by providing transport facilities. Further, these poor, rural women need good quality, affordable services when they arrive at the hospital. An effective community-based, advocacy organisation could easily organise transport for transferring patients to hospitals, provided the community actively participates. In addition, it can arrange an interest-free loan from a community-operated fund to meet urgent needs of money for hospital treatment. There are precedents for this around the world, which in fact, fall within the tradition of the Friendly Societies that once operated in Britain. What I am proposing here is a form of local insurance initiative in which a community-operated fund is created by seeking a very small amount of contribution from the community and a subsidy from NGOs and international donors.

The matter of financial resources is crucial. If the State provides financial resources from the revenue budget for modern biomedical practices, it must allocate some resources to improve indigenous birth practices. But, at the same time, it is also important for the State to restrain itself from having control over the issue. It means that community-based organisation for women's health must run autonomously and without professional interventions. This does not imply second-rate, non-expert organisations. Rather, such women's health organisations will have their own system of accountability to the women of the village. Political advocacy will be required to re-orientate both the State and international funding agencies to support indigenous birthing.

Re-organisation of Hospital Services

The propositions for improving cosmopolitan obstetric practices are based on the principles stated in the Ottawa Charter (World Health Organisation, 1986) for reorienting health services. It stipulates concerted action of government, non-governmental organisations, local authorities, educationists, families, industry and the media to organise health services. The mandate for improving the health sector will assist in organising hospital obstetric services in Bangladesh for rural, poor women. A few issues are of immediate concern: upgrading the THC with comprehensive obstetric care; providing gender and culturally sensitive environment; sensitising biomedical professionals; and improving the service quality.

As childbirth is considered a normal event, it is important not to encourage normal deliveries in hospitals. However, in the event of women needing hospital obstetric care, the Dutch model[1] (van Alten, 1984), which essentially favours home birth, suggests the possibility of using medical indications for hospital confinement. Some of the suggested criteria for hospital admission, such as age, previous history of complications and timing of labour onset are still debatable. However, this model does establish a culture of justifying why it is necessary to go to hospital. It also contributes to a culture of assuming the normality of home, or indigenous, birth. On the other hand, use of such criteria in selecting hospital confinement will minimise the chances of fatal consequences and unnecessary travelling during labour.

The upgrading of the THCs with comprehensive obstetric care is need now. The doctors and nurses performing caesarean section or assisted vaginal delivery need to be proficient and skilled in managing it. In case of grave complications, where further skills are required, an arrangement should be made to seek assistance of the senior consultants posted in the Medical College Hospital or District Hospital. Under no circumstances should patients be required to move from one hospital to another. If THCs provide comprehensive obstetric care, it will reduce the costs of treatment, and problems of distance, and spatial configuration of larger hospital.

This study has highlighted the need for hospitals to develop processes that address the issues of demedicalising birth and deprofessionalising medical professions. I do not encourage normal birth to happen in hospitals, however, when it occurs, women's active participation in birth is acknowledged underscoring the importance of the demedicalisation. The deprofessionalisation of medical professions should be stressed in order to abolish the dominance of monopolistic, authoritative knowledge of biomedical professionals. Doctors should employ their skills and expertise, but encouraging women to use their own embodied knowledge and providing full medical information in an understandable manner make birthing participatory and reduce the gap in knowledge between biomedical professionals and women. Interpersonal relationship between biomedical professionals and rural women can be improved by continuing tolerant, sympathetic conversation and using local dialects as much as possible. These issues need serious consideration in order to create participatory environment in hospital birth practices.

To make hospital environment user friendly, gender and cultural issues are required to be addressed. In labour room, maintaining privacy, providing emotional support, changing labour tables to normal sized beds or floor beds, encouraging women's preferred birthing positions and arranging *en suite* toilets are all necessary. Issues of privacy also need to be considered in obstetric wards during patient examinations. To accommodate a male doctor's presence and assistance during patient examination or child delivery, a comfortable interpersonal relationship between women and male doctors is particularly essential. Information corners are required to be located in convenient places providing necessary information in an understandable manner with pictorial demonstrations for people who cannot read. Even small changes will make the hospital environment more receptive to poor rural women and their attendants and provide them with dignity.

Sensitising biomedical professionals, including nurses, is a critical task that should be initiated at the start in their education. Medical and nursing curricula must stress on the issue of demedicalising birth events and treating patients as a whole human being with physical, psychological, emotional and financial needs. It should also stipulate improving hospital service quality and maintaining congenial relationships with colleagues and hospital staff. For this, it is necessary for the curriculum to extend beyond medical textbooks to include the realities of people's lives, hospital organisation and the rural contexts. The history of biomedicine, indigenous medicine and midwifery, the social roots of deaths and diseases and the politics of health should become important features in medical education. In addition, medical and nursing education should also stress on exposing medical students and nurses to indigenous birth practices by arranging their visits to indigenous archives maintained in community-based women organisations. In order to create humane, pro-poor, pro-people medical curricula a multidisciplinary team of educators is essential.

The improvement of service quality in hospitals can be sustained through quality assurance programmes that not only monitor service provision through hospital statistics, but also scrutinise activities through frequent, small-scale research. In other words, quality assurance should evaluate hospital processes as well as service outcomes. The quality assurance system is built up in such way that will include public accountability of health care and health care professionals (Wagner, 1995). Moreover, the focus of the quality assurance programme is to ensure technological aspects of medical care, to maintain aseptic practices in hospitals and to ascertain the use of hospital-available drugs and other hospital facilities. In this regard, short training in quality improvement can be arranged for both senior and junior doctors and nurses in hospitals. It is also crucial to ensure that pharmaceutical companies cannot directly influence medical doctors and access hospital wards. Their contact with doctors should be limited to formal meetings, seminars and conferences. Maintaining congenial and collaborative relationship between doctors and nurses and seniors and juniors is necessary to reduce predicaments in managing poor patients and to minimise their stress and workload. The success of quality assurance will depend on the absolute commitment of doctors, nurses and hospital administrators that will eventually improve service quality and outcome of treatment, and reduce hospital expenditures and costs of treatment borne by patients.

As the service quality is affected by corrupt practices, an immediate concern is to focus on how to rectify this. In this regard, transparency of decisions or acts including expenditures, decentralisation of power and job accountability may help. Transparency of decisions may be enhanced by the involvement of government, NGOs, civil society and women organisations in hospital boards and executives. Delegating power to peripheral hospitals and assigning some responsibilities to the private sectors, for example, drug supply, laboratories, blood bank and ambulance services are likely to lessen corruptive practices in hospitals. Effective supervision and strict evaluation of job performance may enhance accountability and reduce corruption. More important is the participation of the civil society to access information of hospital activities, and to voice and act in order to ensure better care.

Degovernmentalisaton of the State

The State is overpowered by influencing policy formulation, manipulating financial resources and implementing maternal health care programmes. In order to degovernmentalise the State, the involvement of different groups including NGOs, civil society, women organisations, private enterprises, politicians and donors should be involved in policy decisions and resource allocations. At programme levels, the activities are essential to be shared with NGOs, women organisations and private sectors. Delegating and sharing activities at different levels will minimise power manipulations of the government sectors. At the same time, transparency of acts or decisions should readily be available to enhance the accountability to public.

Democratisation of Health Policy

The bottom-line of maternal health is socio-economic. The narrow, Essential Obstetric Care (EsOC) approach of Safe Motherhood Initiatives does not suffice to address maternal health. In this context, any recommendations to improve the lot of rural, birthing women in Bangladesh must include a policy dimension. The Ottawa Charter (World Health Organisation, 1986), on which the recommendations arising from this study are based, draws on public health policy that emphasises the integration of health into the agenda of all sectors leading to health, income and greater equity. This results in policy making and programme implementation requiring the concerted efforts and political commitments of all government sectors from macro to micro level, from donors to NGOs, from civil society to political parties and from women's organisations to individual woman and man to improve maternal health status and access to better maternal health care in Bangladesh. Even with all such efforts to improve maternal health and health care, it is important to add-in specific acknowledgement of indigenous birth practices in healthy public policy to create pro-women birthing care and opportunities.

Support at International Level

Organising international support to improve maternal health is essential not only in securing financial assistance but also in collaborating with lobbying groups to articulate maternal health and health care needs, particularly in developing countries like Bangladesh. It is important to create pressure at international level and national level in order to bring changes in the strategies of the Safe Motherhood Initiatives from a narrow focus on EsOC to a broader focus in improving maternal health and health care. The commitment of the Safe Motherhood Initiatives should be: to improve socio-economic status; to facilitate education programmes; and to provide accessible and culturally sensitive, comprehensive reproductive health care for poor, rural women. An international monitoring team is required, not from the World Bank or WHO, but from women's organisations, scholars and activists in order to monitor changes in policies and programme implementations and the outcome of global agendas at national levels. This monitoring team should have linkage with community women's health organisations not only to acknowledge indigenous knowledge of birth, but also to do research for further development and to share this knowledge at global levels. Such efforts will bring changes at grassroots levels where rural, poor women desperately need sensitive health care.

Modern medicine as well as cosmopolitan obstetrics have triumphed the West. Nevertheless, even in the West, women have created options for alternative birthing care. In Bangladesh, like many developing countries, cosmopolitan obstetrics have yet to devour indigenous birth practices. Indigenous birth practices are challenged at national and global levels with an attempt to introduce 'cosmopolitically' packaged obstetric care by displacing the former. Whatever be the policy implications, cosmopolitan obstetrics is not the ultimate solution to ensure better maternal health. Women need hospital obstetric care only for birth complications. Indigenous birthing care, shared and supported by women is able to manage normal birth. What is crucial to improve maternal heath in Bangladesh is to eradicate the roots of its causes – poverty, illiteracy, poor housing, poor environment, inadequate access to quality health care, gender disparity and many more issues.

Here, I tell and retell birth stories not only to reveal and reaffirm women's experiences, but also to give voice to women, to reinstate their indigenous knowledge of birth and to reinforce the power of giving birth. I began the research with the aim of exploring why and in what ways rural, poor women in Bangladesh adhere to indigenous birth practices and, concurrently, resist cosmopolitan obstetrics. My research demonstrates that rural, poor women do adhere to indigenous birth practices and, they do resist cosmopolitan obstetrics. A Foucauldian perspective has revealed the layered structures of power enforcing poor women's silence and working in consent to maintain a hierarchical, modern, medical system to the detriment of individual women's lives and to the loss of diversity of health knowledge. These stories open up new horizons to protect childbirth from the rampant charge of modernity and social forces, and to organise women and their sympathisers all over the world to speak up and work for the women to ensure their good health and health care.

Note

[1] Symptoms of toxaemia; cephalopelvic disproportion; no previous history of complications; nulliparous woman older than 35 years; multiparous woman more than 45 years; women not in good health; labour before 37 weeks or after 42 weeks.

References

Afsana, K. (1994). *Perceptions of mother about maternal health care and their utilisation of health services in WHDP*. (BRAC research report: Health studies). Dhaka: BRAC.

Afsana, K. & Mahmud S.N. (1998).*Validation of baseline information of Reproductive Health and Disease Control Programme*. (BRAC research report: Health studies). Dhaka: BRAC.

Afsana, K. & Rashid, S. F. (2001). The challenges of meeting rural women's needs in delivery care. *Reproductive Health Matters, 9 (18)*, 79-89.

—— (2000). *Discoursing birthing care. Experiences from Bangladesh*. Dhaka: The University Press Limited.

Ahmed, R. (2001). The emergence of the Bengal Muslims. In R. Ahmed (Ed.), *Understanding the Bengal Muslims. Interpretative Essays*. Dhaka: The University Press Limited, 1-25.

Ahmed, I. (2002). 'Macro-micro linkages: Critical issues'. Paper presented at the UNDP Workshop on the Assessing Linkages between Micro and Macro Level Issues, UNDP Delhi, India.

—— (2001). Globalisation, State and Political Process in South Asia. In A.R. Khan (Ed.), *Globalisation and non-traditional security in South Asia*. Colombo: Regional Centre for Strategic Studies, 32-70.

—— (1999*)*. *On securing women's security: Perspectives from South Asia*. Plenary lecture presented at the International Conference on the Women and Peace: War, Resistance and Justice, Pennsylvania, USA.

—— (1995). On feminist methodology: Can *mohilas* speak? *Theoretical Perspectives, 2 (1)*, 1-14.

Akhter, H.A., Rahman, M.H., Mannan, I., Elahi, M.E. & Khan, A.K.Z. (1995). *Review of performance of trained TBAs*. Dhaka: BIRPERHT.

Alauddin, M. (1986). Maternal mortality in rural Bangladesh: The Tangail district. *Studies in Family Planning, 17 (1)*, 13-21.

Annadale, E. (1996). Professional defenses: Medical students' perceptions of medical malpractice. *International Journal of Health Services, 26 (4)*, 751-775.

Anonymous. (Personal communication, January 20, 2001a).

——, (Personal communication, May 11-12, 2001b).

——, (Personal communication, August 24-25, 2001c).

Altheide, D.L. & Johnson, J.M. (1994). Criteria for assessing interpretive validity in qualitative research. In N.K. Denzin & Y.S. Lincoln (Eds.), *Handbook of qualitative research*. London: Sage, 485-499.

Bangladesh Bureau of Statistics, (2000). *Statistical pocketbook of Bangladesh 2000*. Dhaka: Ministry of Planning, Government of the People's Republic of Bangladesh.

_____ (1999). *Health situation and health care expenditures in Bangladesh*. Dhaka: Ministry of Planning, Government of the People's Republic of Bangladesh.

Bangladesh Fourth Population and Health Project. (1999). Dhaka: People's Republic of Bangladesh and the Donor Consortium.

Barfield, T. (1996). *Blackwell Dictionary of Anthropology* (Ist ed.). Oxford: Blackwell Publishers. Retrieved October 14, 2002, from http:/www.davis-floyd.com/art_index.html.

Barkat, A., Helali, J., Faisal., A.J. & Bose, M.L. (1995). *Knowledge, attitude and practices relevant to the utilisation of emergency obstetric care services in Bangladesh: A formative study*, Dhaka: University Research Corporation.

Barker, K.K. (1998). A ship upon a stormy sea: The medicalization of pregnancy, *Social Science and Medicine, 47 (8),* 1067-1076.

Becker, A. (1993). *Body, self and society. The view from Fiji*. Philadelphia: University of Pennsylvania Press.

Belle, A. (2002). *Three viewpoints on the praxis and concepts of midwifery: Indian dais, cosmopolitan obstetrics and Japanese seitai*. Retrieved on April 7, 2002, from http://www.bioethics.ws/dais/daicomp.html.

Bhatia, S., Chakravarty, J. & Faruque, A.S.G. (1980). *Indigenous birth practices in rural Bangladesh and their implications for a maternal and child health programme*. Dhaka: International Centre for Diarrhoeal Disease Research, Bangladesh.

Biesele, M. (1997). An ideal of unassisted birth. Hunting, healing and transformation among the Kalahari Ju/'hoansi. In R.E. Davis-Floyd, & C.F. Sargent (Eds.), *Childbirth and authoritative knowledge: Cross-cultural perspectives*. London: University of California Press, 474-492.

Biswas, S., Dasgupta, B. & Sengupta, S. (1968). *Samsad Bengali-English Dictionary* (2nd ed.). Calcutta: Sahitya Samsad.

Blanchet, T. (1991). *Maternal health in rural Bangladesh. An anthropological study on maternal nutrition and birth practices in Nasirnagar, Bangladesh*. Dhaka: Save the Children (USA).

_____ (1988). *Maternal mortality in Bangladesh. Anthropological assessment report*. Dhaka: NORAD.

_____ (1984). *Women, pollution and marginality: Meanings and rituals of birth in rural Bangladesh*. Dhaka: The University Press Limited.

Bloor, M. & Macintosh, J. (1990). Surveillance and concealment: A comparison of techniques of client resistance in therapeutic communities and health visiting. In S. Cunnigham-Burley & N. P. Mckeganey (Eds.), *Readings in medical sociology*. London: Routledge, 159-181.

Bordo, S. (1999). Feminism, Foucault and the politics of the body. In J. Price & M. Shildrick (Eds.), *Feminist theory and the body. A reader*. Edinburgh: Edinburgh University Press, 246-257.

Broom, D.H. (1991). *Damned if we do. Contradictions in women's health care*. North Sydney: Allen & Unwin.

Browner, C. & Press, N. (1997). The production of authoritative knowledge in American prenatal care. In R.E. Davis-Floyd & C.F. Sargent (Eds.), *Childbirth and authoritative knowledge: Cross-cultural perspectives*. London: University of California Press, 113-131.

Chatterjee, P. (1993). *The Nation and its fragments. Colonial and postcolonial histories*. New Jersey: Princeton University Press.

Chawla, J. (2002). Hawa, gola and mother-in-law's big toe: On understanding dais' imagery of the female body. In G. Samuel & S. Rozario (Eds.), *The daughters of Hariti: Childbirth and female healers in South and Southeast Asia*. London & New York: Routledge,147-162.

Chowdhury, A.M.R., Mahbub, A. & Chowdhury, A.S. (2002), Skilled attendance at delivery in Bangladesh: An ethnographic study. *BRAC Research Monograph*. (Serial No. 22). Dhaka: BRAC.

Chowdhury, Z. (1996). *The politics of essential drugs. The making of a successful health strategy: Lessons from Bangladesh*. Dhaka: The University Press Limited.

Cosminsky, S. (1982). Childbirth and change: A Guatemalan study. Health, fertility and birth in Moyamba District, Sierra Leone. In C.P. MacCormack (Ed.), *Ethnography of fertility and birth*. London: Academic Press, 205-229.

Cosslett, T. (1994). *Women writing childbirth. Modern discourses of motherhood*. Manchester: Manchester University Press.

Coulson, J., Carr, C.T., Hutchison, L. & Eagle, D. (1962). *Oxford Illustrated Dictionary* (2nd ed.). London: Book Club Associates.

Cousins, M. & Hussain, A. (1984). *Michel Foucault*. London: MacMillan.

Cranny-Francis, A. (1995). *The body in the text*. Melbourne: Melbourne University Press.

Das, V. (1997). Language and body: Transaction in the construction of pain. In A. Kleinman, V. Das & M. Lock (Eds.), *Social sufferings*. Berkley: University of California Press, 67-92.

Davis-Floyd, R.E. (1994). The technocratic body: American childbirth as cultural expression. *Social Science and Medicine, 38 (8)*, 1125-1140.

_____ (1992). *Birth as an American rite of passage*. Berkley: University of California Press.

_____ (1990). The role of obstetrical rituals in the resolution of cultural anomaly. *Social Science and Medicine, 31 (2)*, 175-189.

Davis-Floyd, R.E. & Sargent, C. (1997). Introduction: The anthropology of birth. In R.E. Davis-Floyd & C.F. Sargent (Eds.), *Childbirth and authoritative knowledge: Cross-cultural perspectives*. London: University of California Press,1-51.

Denzin, N.K. (1997). *Interpretive ethnography: Ethnographic practices for the 21st century*. London: Sage.

_____ (1994). The art and politics of interpretation. In N.K. Denzin & Y.S. Lincoln (Eds.), *Handbook of qualitative research*. London: Sage, 500-515.

Doyal, L. (1995). *What makes women sick. Gender and the political economy of health*. London: MacMillan Press.

_____ (1979). *The political economy of health*. London: Pluto Press.

Dunn, F.L. (1976). Traditional Asian medicine and cosmopolitan medicine as adaptive systems. In C. Leslie (Ed.), *Asian medical systems. A comparative study*. London: University of California Press, 133-158.

Dutt, D. (1975). In politics. In S. Kohli (Ed.), *Corruption in India*. New Delhi: Chetana Publications, 77-95.

Eaoton, R.M. (2001). Who are the Bengal Muslims? Conversion and Islamization in Bengal. In R. Ahmed (Ed.), *Understanding Bengal Muslims. Interpretative essays*. Dhaka: The University Press Limited, 26-51.

Ehrenreich, B. & English, D. (1973). *Witches, midwives and nurses. A history of women healers*. New York: The Feminist Press.

Favre-Saada, J. (1980). *Deadly words. Witchcraft in the Bocage*. Cambridge: Cambridge University Press.

Fisher, S. (1991). A discourse of the social: Medical talk/power talk/ oppositional talk?. *Discourse & Society, 2 (2),* 157-182.

Foster, G.M., & Anderson, B.G. (1978). *Medical Anthropology.* New York: Alfred A. Knopf.

Foucault, M. (1991a). Questions of method. In G. Burchell, C. Gordon & P. Miller (Eds.), *The Foucault effect. Studies in governmentality.* Chicago: The University of Chicago Press, 73-86.

_____ (1991b). Governmentality. In G. Burchell, C. Gordon & P. Miller (Eds.), *The Foucault effect. Studies in governmentality.* Chicago: The University of Chicago Press, 87-104.

_____ (1987a). Space, knowledge and power. In P. Rabinow (Ed.), *The Foucault reader.* New York: Penguin Books, 239-256.

_____ (1987b). Truth and power. In P. Rabinow (Ed.), *The Foucault reader.* New York: Penguin Books, 51-75.

_____ (1982a). Power and truth. In H. Dreyfus & P. Rabinow (Eds.), *Michel Foucault: Beyond structuralism and hermeneutics.* Sussex: The Harvester Press, 184-207.

_____ (1982b). The subject and power. In H. Dreyfus & P. Rabinow (Eds.), *Michel Foucault: Beyond structuralism and hermeneutics.* Sussex: The Harvester Press, 208-226.

_____ (1980a). Two lectures. In C. Gordon (Ed.), *Power/knowledge: Selected interviews & other writings.* New York: Pantheon Books, 78-108.

_____ (1980b). The Politics of health in the eighteenth century. In C. Gordon (Ed.), *Power/knowledge: Selected interviews & other writings.* New York: Pantheon Books, 166-182.

_____ (1978). *The history of sexuality.* Volume 1: *An introduction.* (R Hurley, Trans.). Harmondsworth: Penguin (Original work published in 1976).

_____ (1977). *Discipline and punishment: The birth of the prison.* (A. Sheridan, Trans.). New York: Penguin (Original work published in 1975).

_____ (1973). *The birth of the Clinic. An archaeology of medical perception.* (A. Sheridan, Trans.). London: Routledge (Original work published in 1963).

Freidson, E. (1971). Professions and the occupational principle. In E. Freidson (Ed.), *The professions and their prospects.* London: Sage Publications, 19-38.

_____ (1970). *Profession of medicine.* New York: Dodd, Mead.

Fromm, E., (1955). *The sane society.* New York: Henry Holy and Company.

Ganatra, B.R., Coyaji, K.J. & Rao, V.N. (1998). Too far, too little, too late: A community-based case-control study of maternal mortality in rural West Maharashtra, India. *Bulletin of World Health Organization, 76 (6),* 591-598.

Gardner, K. (1991). *Songs at the River's Edge: Stories from a Bangladeshi Village*. Delhi: Rupa & Co.

Gaskin, I.M. (1990). *Spiritual Midwifery* (3rd ed.). Summertown, Tennessee: The Book Publishing Company.

Gazi, R. (1998). *Barriers to emergency obstetric care in rural Bangladesh*. (BRAC Research Report, Health Studies). Dhaka: BRAC.

Good, B.J. (1997). *Medicine, rationality and experience*. Cambridge: Cambridge University Press.

Goodburn, E.A., Chowdhury, M., Gazi, R., Marshall, T., Graham, W. & Karim, F. (1994). *An investigation into the nature and determinants of maternal morbidity related to delivery and the puerperium in rural Bangladesh*. Dhaka: BRAC.

Goodburn, E.A., Gazi, R. & Chowdhury, M. (1995). Beliefs and practices regarding delivery and postpartum maternal morbidity in rural Bangladesh, *Studies in Family Planning, 26 (1)*, 22-32.

Goodburn, E.A., Chowdhury, M., Gazi, R., Marshall, T. & Graham, W. (2000). Training traditional birth attendants in clean delivery does not prevent postpartum infection. *Studies in Family Planning, 15 (4)*, 394-399.

Graham, H. & Oakley, A. (1981). Competing ideologies of reproduction: Medical and material perspectives on pregnancy. In H. Roberts (Ed.), *Women, health and reproduction*. London: Routledge & Kegan Paul, 50-74.

Greenhalgh, S. (1995). Anthropology theorizes reproduction: Intigrating practice, political economic, and feminist perspectives. In S. Greenhalgh (Ed.), *Situating Fertility: Anthropology and Demographic Inquiry*. London: Cambridge University Press, 3-28.

Guba, E.G. & Lincoln, Y.S. (1994). Competing paradigms in qualitative research. In N.K. Denzin & Y.S. Lincoln (Eds.), *Handbook of qualitative research*. London: Sage, 105-177.

Gupta, A., Choudhury, B.R., Balachandran, I., Vincent, P., Khanna, R., Nissim, R., et al. (1997). *Touch me, touch-me-not. Women, plants and healing*. New Delhi: Kali for Women.

Gupta, B. (1976). Indigenous medicine in nineteenth and twentieth-century Bengal. In C. Leslie (Ed.), *Asian medical systems. A comparative study*. London: University of California Press, 368-377.

Hahn, R.A. & Gaines, A.D. (1985). Among the physicians: Encounter, exchange and transformation. In R.A. Hahn and A.D. Gaines (Eds.), *Physicians of western medicine. Anthropological approaches to theory and practice*. Boston: D. Reidel Publishing Company, 3-21.

Haque, Y.A. & Mostafa, G. (1993). *A review of emergency obstetric care functions of selected facilities in Bangladesh*. Dhaka: UNICEF.

Hudson-Rodd, N. (1994). Public health: People participating in the creation of healthy places. *Public Health Nursing, 11 (2)*, 119-126.

Hunt, L. (1998). Woman-to-woman support: Lessons from an Australian case story. *Patient Education and Counseling, 33*, 257-265.

Illich, I. (1977). Disabling professions. In I. Illich, I.K. Zola, J. Caplan, & H.Shaiken (Eds.). *Disabling professions*. London: Marion Boyars, 11-39.

_____ (1976). *Medical nemesis: The exploration of health*. New York: Pantheon Books.

Irigaray, L. (1991). Women-amongst-themselves: Creating a woman-to-woman sociality. In M. Whitford (Ed.), *The Irigaray reader*. Oxford: Blackwell, 190-197.

Jahan, K. & Hossain, M. (1998). *Bangladesh national nutrition survey of 1995-96*. Dhaka: Dhaka Institute of Nutrition and Food Science, Dhaka University.

Jansick, V.J. (1994). The dance of qualitative research design. In N.K. Denzin & Y.S. Lincoln (Eds.), *Handbook of qualitative research*. London: Sage, 209-219.

Jeffery, P., Jeffery, R. & Lyon, A. (1989). *Labour pains and labour power: Women and childbearing in India*. London: Zed Books.

Jeffery, R. & Jeffery, P.M. (1993). Traditional birth attendants in rural North India: The social organization of childbearing. In S. Lindenbaum & M. Lock (Eds.), *Knowledge, Power and Practice*. Berkley: University of California Press, 7-31.

Jirojwong, S. (1996). Health beliefs and the use of antenatal care among pregnant women in Southern Thailand. In P.L. Rice & L. Manderson (Eds.), *Maternity and reproductive health in Asian societies*. The Netherlands: Harwood Academic Publishers, 61-82.

Johnstone, M.J. (2002). Poor working conditions and the capacity of nurses to provide moral care. *Contemporary Nurse, 12 (1)*, 9-15.

Jones, S. (1985). Depth interviewing. In R. Walker (Ed.), *Applied qualitative research*. Aldershot: Gower, 45-55.

Jordan, B. (1997). Authoritative knowledge and its construction. In R.E. Davis-Floyd & C.F. Sargent (Eds.), *Childbirth and authoritative knowledge: Cross-cultural perspectives*. London: University of California Press, 55-79.

_____ (1993). *Birth in four cultures: A crosscultural investigation of childbirth in Yucatan, Holland, Sweden, and the United States* (4th ed. rev. & exp. by R. Davis-Floyd). Prospect Heights, IL: Waveland.

Jordan, B. (1989). Cosmopolitical obstetrics: Some insights from the training of traditional midwives. *Social Science and Medicine*, 28 (9), 925-944.

_____ (1983). *Birth in four cultures*. London: Eden Press.

Juncker, T., Khan, M.H. & Ahmed, S. (1996). 'Interventions in obstetric care: Lessons learned from Abhoynagar' (Working Paper No. 124). Dhaka: International Centre for Diarrhoeal Disease Research, Bangladesh.

Juncker, T. & Khanum, P.A. (1997). 'Obstetric complications: The health care-seeking process before admission at the hospital in rural Bangladesh' (Working Paper No. 132). Dhaka: International Centre for Diarrhoeal Disease Research, Bangladesh.

Kakar, D.N. (1980). *Dais: The traditional birth attendants in village India*. Delhi: New Asian Publishers.

Kaufert, P.A. & O'Neil, J.D. (1993). Analysis of a dialogue on risks in childbirth. In S. Lindenbaum & M. Lock (Eds.), *Knowledge, power and practice*. Berkley: University of California Press, 32-54.

_____ (1990). Cooptation and control: The reconstruction of birth. *New Series, 4 (4)*, 427-442.

Kay, M.A. (1982). Writing an ethnography of birth. In A. Margarita (Ed.), *Anthropology of Human Birth*. Philadelphia: FA Davis Company, 1-24.

Khan, A.R., Jahan, F.A. & Begum, S.F. (1986), Maternal mortality in rural Bangladesh: The Jamalpur District. *Studies in Family Planning, 17 (1)*, 7-12.

Khan, M.S.H., Kanam, S.T., Nahar, S., Nasrin, T. & Rahman, A.P.M.S. (2000). *Review of availability and use of emergency obstetric care (EOC) services in Bangladesh*. Dhaka: Associates for Community and Population Research.

Khuse, H. (1997). *Caring: Nurses, women and ethics*. Oxford: Blackwell Publisher.

Killingsworth, J.R., Hossain, N., Hedrick-Wong, Y., Thomas, S., Rahman, A. & Begum, T. (1999). Unofficial fees in Bangladesh: Price, equity and institutional issues. *Health Policy and Management, 14 (2)*, 152-163.

Kitzinger, S. (2002). *Birth your way. Choosing birth at home or in a birth centre*. London: Dorling Kindersley.

_____ (1997). Authoritative touch in childbirth: A cross-cultural approach. In R.E. Davis-Floyd & C.F. Sargent (Eds.), *Childbirth and authoritative knowledge: Cross-cultural perspectives*. London: University of California Press, 209-232.

_____ (1991). *Home birth and other alternatives to hospital*. London: Dorling Kindersley.

Kitzinger, S. (1982). The social context of birth: Some comparisons between childbirth in Jamaica and Britain. In C.P. MacCormack (Ed.), *Ethnography of fertility and birth*. London: Academic Press, 181-203.

Kleinman, A. (1995). *Writing at margin: Discourses between anthropology and medicine*. Berkley: University of California Press.

_____ (1986). Illness meaning and illness behaviour. In S. McHugh & T.M. Vallis (Eds.), *Illness behaviour. A multidisciplinary model*. London: Plenum Press, 149-160.

_____ (1980). *Patients and healers in the context of culture. An exploration of the borderland between anthropology, medicine and psychiatry*. London: University of California Press.

Koblinsky, M.A., Campbell, O.M.R. & Harlow, S.D. (1993). Mother and more: A broader perspective on women's health. In M.A. Koblinsky, J. Timyan & J. Gay (Eds.), *The health of women: A global perspective*. Boulder: Westview Press, 33-61.

Kohli, S. (1975). The psychology of corruption. In S. Kohli (Ed.), *Corruption in India*. New Delhi: Chetana Publications, 32-38.

Konner, M. (1987). *Becoming a doctor: A journey of initiation in medical school*. New York: Viking.

Kothari, M.L. & Mehta, L.A. (1988). Violence in modern medicine. In A. Nandy (Ed.), *Science, hegemony and violence. A requiem for modernity*. Delhi: Oxford University Press, 167-210.

Laderman, C. (1982). Giving birth in a Malay village. In A. Margarita (Ed.), *Anthropology of human birth*, Philadelphia: FA Davis Company, 81-100.

Lawrence, J.V. (1992). *Architecture, power and national identity*. New Haven: Yale University Press.

Lazaraus, E. (1997). What do women want? Issues of choice, control and class in American pregnancy and childbirth. In R.E. Davis-Floyd & C.F. Sargent (Eds.), *Childbirth and authoritative knowledge: Cross-cultural perspectives*. London: University of California Press, 132-158.

_____ (1988). Theoretical considerations for the study of the doctor-patient relationship: Implications of a perinatal study, *New Series, 2 (1)*, 34-58.

Leppard, M. (2000). *Obstetric care in Bangladesh District Hospital: An organizational ethnography*. Unpublished doctoral dissertation. London: London School of Hygiene and Tropical Medicine.

Leslie, C. (1976). Introduction. In C. Leslie (Ed.), *Asian medical systems. A comparative study*. London: University of California Press, 1-17.

Lindenbaum, S. (1979). *Kuru sorcery: Disease and danger in the New Guinea highlands*. Palo Alto, California: Mayfield Pub. Co.

Lock, M. & Scheper-Hughes, N. (1990). A critical-interpretive approach in medical anthropology: rituals and routines of discipline and dissent. In T.M. Johnson & C.F. Sargent (Eds.), *Medical anthropology. A handbook of theory and method*. London: Greenwood Press, 47-72.

MacCormack, C.P. (1982). Health, fertility and birth in Moyamba District, Sierra Leone. In C.P. MacCormack (Ed.), *Ethnography of fertility and birth*. London: Academic Press, 115-139.

Maloney, C., Aziz, K.M.A. & Sarker, P. (1981). *Beliefs and fertility in Bangladesh*. Dhaka: International Centre for Diarrhoeal Disease Research, Bangladesh.

Martin, E. (1990). Science and women's bodies: Forms of anthropological knowledge. In M. Jacobus, E.F. Keller & S. Shuttleworth (Eds.), *Body/politics. Women and the discourse of science*. London: Routledge, 69-82.

_____ (1989).*The woman in the body. A cultural analysis of reproduction*. Buckingham: Open University Press.

McKeown, T. (1989). *The role of medicine. Dream, mirage or nemesis?* Oxford: Basil Blackwell.

Ministry of Finance. (2002). *Bangladesh: A national strategy for economic growth and poverty reduction*. Dhaka: Government of the People's Republic of Bangladesh.

Ministry of Health and Family Welfare. (1998a). *HPSP 1998-2003. Programme implementation plan part I (1998)*. Dhaka: Government of the People's Republic of Bangladesh.

_____ (1998b). *HPSP 1998-2003. Programme implementation plan part II (1998)*. Dhaka: Government of the People's Republic of Bangladesh.

_____ (1998c). *National health policy, 1405 (B.E) 1998*. Dhaka: Government of the People's Republic of Bangladesh.

Mishler, E.G. (1984). *The discourse of medicine: Dialectics of medical interviews*. Norwood: Ablex Publishing.

Mitra, S.N., Ali, M.N., Islam, S., Cross, A. & Saha, T. (1994). *Bangladesh demographic and health survey 1993-94*. Dhaka: NIPORT.

Nandy, A. (1995).*The savage Freud and other essays on possible and retrievable selves. Return from exile*. Delhi: Oxford University Press.

_____ (1990). *At the Edge of Psychology: Essays in Politics and Culture* (2nd ed.). Delhi: Oxford University Press.

Nahar, S. & Costello, A. (1998). The hidden cost of 'free' maternity in Dhaka, Bangladesh. *Health Policy and Planning, 13 (4)*. 417-422.

National Institute for Population Research and Training. (2002). *Preliminary report. Bangladesh maternal health services and maternal mortality survey 2001*. Dhaka: NIPORT and Measure DHS+ORC Macro.

Navarro, V. (2000). Development and quality of life: A critique of Amartya Sen's development as freedom. *International Journal of Health Services, 30 (4)*, 661-674.

_____ (1981). The underdevelopment of health or the health of underdevelopment: An analysis of the distribution of human health resources in Latin America. In V. Navarro (Ed.), *Imperialism, health and medicine*. New York: Baywood Publishing Company, Inc., 15-37.

Navarro, V. & Shi, L. (2001). The political context of social inequalities and health. *International Journal of Health Services, 31 (1)*, 1-21.

O'Neil, J. & Kauffert, P. (1990). The politics of obstetric care: The Inuit experience. In W.P. Handwerker (Ed.), *Births and power: Social change and the politics of reproduction*. London: Westview Press, 53-68.

Oakley, A. (1993). *The essays on women, medicine and health*. Edinburgh: Edinburgh University Press.

_____ (1984). *The captured womb. A history of the medical care of pregnant women*. New York: Basil Blackwell.

_____ (1980). *Women confined. Towards a sociology of childbirth*. Oxford: Martin Robertson.

_____ (1979). *Becoming a mother*. Oxford: Martin Robertson.

Olsen, V. (1994). Feminism and models of qualitative research. In N.K. Denzin & Y.S. Lincoln (Eds.), *Handbook of qualitative research*. London: Sage, 158-174.

Patel, T. (1999). The precious few: Women's agency, household progressions and fertility in Rajasthan village. *Journal of Comparative Family Studies, 30 (3)*, 429-457.

Paul, B.K. (1983). A note on the hierarchy of health facilities in Bangladesh. *Social Science and Medicine, 17 (3)*, 189-191.

Phillips, D.R. (1990). *Health and health care in the third world*. New York: Longman, Scientific & Technical.

Phillips, D.R. & Verhasselt, Y. (1994). Introduction: Health and development. In D.R. Phillips & Y. Verhasselt (Eds.), *Health and development*. London: Routledge, 3-32.

Porter, M. (1990). Professional-client relationships and women's reproductive health care. In S. Cunnigham-Burley & N. P. Mckeganey (Eds.), *Readings in medical sociology*. London: Routledge, 182-212.

Porter, S. (1999). Working with doctors. In G. Wilkinson & M. Miers (Eds.), *Power and nursing practice. Sociology and nursing practice series.* London: Macmillan, 97-110.

Quaiyum, M. A., Ahmed, S., Islam, A. & Khanum, P. A. (1999). 'Strategies for ensuring referral and linkage for essential obstetric care: A review'. (ICDDR,B Working Paper Special Publication). Dhaka: International Centre for Diarrhoeal Disease Research, Bangladesh.

Ram, K. (2001). Modernity and the midwife: Contestations over a subaltern figure, South India. In L.H. Connor & G. Samuel (Eds.), *Healings powers and modernity. Traditional medicine, shamanism and science in Asian societies.* Westport, Connecticut: Bergin and Garvey, 64-84.

Reynolds, P.C. (1991). *Stealing fire: The atomic bomb as symbolic body.* Palo Alto, California: Iconic Anthropology Press.

Richman, J. (1987). *Medicine and health.* London: Longman.

Rose-Ackerman, S. (1999). *Corruption and government. Causes, consequences and reform.* Cambridge: Cambridge University Press.

_____ (1978). *Corruption. A study in political economy.* London: Academic Press.

Rothman, B.K. (1982). *In labour. Women and power in the birthplace.* London: W.W. Norton & Company.

Rozario, S. (2002). The healer on the margins: The *dai* in rural Bangladesh. In S. Rozario & G. Samuel (Eds.), *The daughters of Hariti: Childbirth and female healers in South and Southeast Asia.* London & New York: Routledge, 130-146.

_____ (1998). The *dai* and the doctor: discourses on women's reproductive health in rural Bangladesh. In K. Ram & M. Jolly (Eds.), *Maternities and modernities: Colonial and postcolonial experiences in Asia and Pacific.* London: Cambridge University Press, 144-176.

_____ (1995). *Dai* and midwives: The renegotiation of the status of birth attendants in contemporary Bangladesh. In J. Hatcher & C. Vlassoff (Eds.), *The female client and the health-care provider.* Ottawa: International Development Research Centre, 91-112.

_____ (1992). *Purity and communal boundaries. Women and social change in a Bangladeshi village.* North Sydney: Allen & Unwin.

Rozario, S. & Samuel, G. (2002). Tibetan and Indian ideas of birth pollution: Similarities and contrasts. In S. Rozario & G. Samuel (Eds.), *The daughters of Hariti: Childbirth and female healers in South and Southeast Asia.* London & New York: Routledge, 182-208.

Sanders, D. & Carver, R. (1985). *The struggle for health. Medicine and the politics of underdevelopment.* London: MacMillan.

REFERENCES

Sargent, C.F. (1990). The politics of birth: Cultural dimensions of pain, virtue, and control among the Bariba of Benin. In W.P. Handwerker (Ed.), *Births and power: Social change and the politics of reproduction*. London: Westview Press, 69-79.

_____ (1989). *Maternity, medicine and power: Reproductive decisions in urban Benin*. Berkley: University of California Press.

_____ (1989). Women's role and women healers in contemporary rural and urban Benin. In C.S. McClain (Ed.), *Women as healers. Cross-cultural perspectives*. London: Rutgers University Press, 204-218.

_____ (1982). Solitary confinement: Birth practices among the Bariba of the People's Republic of Benin. In A. Margarita (Ed.), *Anthropology of human birth*. Philadelphia: FA Davis Company, 193-219.

Sawicki, J. (1991). *Disciplining Foucault: Feminism, power, and the body*. New York: Routledge.

Schulz, R. & Johnson, A.C. (1990). *Management of hospitals and health services. Strategic issues and performance* (3rd ed.). Baltimore: The C.V. Mosby Company.

Sesia, P.M. (1997). "Women come here on their own when they need to": Prenatal care, authoritative knowledge, and maternal health in Oaxaca. In R.E. Davis-Floyd & C.F. Sargent (Eds.), *Childbirth and authoritative knowledge: Cross-cultural perspectives*. London: University of California Press, 397-420.

Shostak, M. (1981). *Nisa: The life and words of a Kung woman*. Cambridge. Massachusetts: Harvard University Press.

Smith, D.E. (1987). *The everyday world as problematic. A feminist sociology*. Boston: Northeastern University Press.

Somjee, G. (1991). Social change in the nursing profession in India. In P. Holden & J. Littlewood (Eds.), *Anthropology in Nursing*. London: Routledge, 31-55.

Sundari, T.K. (1992). The untold story: How health care systems in developing countries contribute to maternal mortality. *International Journal of Health Services, 22 (3)*, 513-528.

Tew, M. (1990). *Safer childbirth? A critical history of maternity care*. London: Chapman and Hall.

Thaddeus, S. & Maine, D. (1994). Too far to walk: Maternal mortality in context. *Social Science and Medicine, 38 (8)*, 1091-1110.

Thomas, S., Killingsworth, J.R. & Acharya, S. (1998). User fees, self-selection and the poor in Bangladesh. *Health Policy and Planning, 13 (1)*, 50-58.

Trevanthan, W.R. (1997). An evolutionary perspective on authoritative knowledge about birth. In R.E. Davis-Floyd & C.F. Sargent (Eds.), *Childbirth and authoritative knowledge: Cross-cultural perspectives*. London: University of California Press, 80-88.

Turner, B.S. (1987). *Medical power and social knowledge*. London: Sage Publications.

Tyler, S.A. (1986). Postmodern ethnography: From the document of the occult to occult document. In J. Clifford & G.E. Marcus (Eds.), *Writing culture: The poetics and politics of ethnography*. Berkley: University of California Press, 122-140.

UNICEF. (1993a). *Emergency obstetric care: Intervention for the reduction of maternal mortality*. Dhaka: Obstetrical and Gynecological Society of Bangladesh.

_____ (1993b). *State of the world's children*. Oxford and New York: Oxford University Press.

Unnithan-Kumar, M. (2002). Midwives and other women: Agency, emotions and the politics of healing in Rajasthan, North West India. In S. Rozario & G. Samuel (Eds.), *The daughters of Hariti: Childbirth and female healers in South and Southeast Asia*. London & New York: Routledge, 109-129.

van Alten, D. (1984). *Obstetric care in the Netherlands*. Amsterdam: Academisch Medisch Centrum.

van Mannen, J. (1988). *Tales of the field: On writing ethnography*. Chicago: The University of Chicago Press.

Vivoni-Farge, E. (2002). The architecture of power: From the neoclassical to modernism in the architecture of Puerto Rico, 1900-1950. *Aris, 3 (1)*, Retrieved on November 20, 2002, from http://www.cmu.edu/ARIS_3/vivoni/vivoni_intro.html.

Wagner, M. (1997). Confessions of a Dissident. In R.E. Davis-Floyd & C.F. Sargent (Eds.), *Childbirth and authoritative knowledge: Cross-cultural perspectives*. London: University of California Press, 366-396.

_____ (1995). A global witch-hunt. *The Lancet, 346 (8981)*, 1020-1023.

_____ (1994). *Pursuing the birth machine. The search for appropriate birth technology*. Camperdown, NSW: Ace Graphics.

Wagner, M., Chin, V.V.P., Peters, C.J., Drexler, B. & Newman, L.A. (1989). A comparison of early and delayed induction of labour with spontaneous rupture of membranes at term. *Obstetrics and Gynaecology, 74 (July)*, 93-97.

Weedon, C. (1987). *Feminist practice and poststructuralist theory*. Oxford: Basil Blackwell.

Whittaker, A. (2000). *Intimate knowledge. Women and their health in North-East Thailand*. New South Wales: Allen & Unwin.

Wilsford, D. (1991). *Doctors and the state. The politics of health care in France and the United States*. London: Duke University Press.

World Health Organisation. (1999). *Reduction of maternal mortality. A joint statement. WHO/UNFPA/UNICEF/World Bank Statement*. Geneva: WHO.

_____ (1996). *Care in normal birth: a practical guide*. Geneva: WHO.

_____ (1986)*Ottawa charter for health promotion*. Ottawa: Canadian Public Health Association.

World Bank Report. (2003). *Bangladesh Economy*. Retrieved January 12, 2003 from http:/www.worldbank.org/data/countrydata/aag/bg_aag.pdf.

_____ (1999). Review of the Health and Population Sector Program: Baseline Service Delivery Survey, Bangladesh. Unpublished manuscript. Dhaka: World Bank.

York, G. (1987). *The high price of health. A patient's guide to the hazards of medical politics*. Toronto: James Lorimer & Company.

Zola, I.K. (1977). Healthism and disabling medicalization. In I. Illich, I.K. Zola, J. Caplan & H. Shaiken (Eds.), *Disabling professions*. London: Marion Boyars, 41-68.

Index

abortion (miscarriage), 112, 144
Acharya, S., 231
Afsana, K., 1, 5-8, 63, 109, 159, 162, 172, 219
agrarian society, 5
Ahmed, I., 1, 13, 16, 169, 194, 219
Ahmed, R., 219
Ahmed, S., 7-8, 226, 230
Akhter, H.A., 219
Alauddin, M., 219
Ali, M.N., 5, 228
allopathy, 20
Alma Ata Declaration, 196
Altheide, D.L., 8, 220
ambulance service, 22, 215
anaemia, 5
Anderson, B.G., 163, 188, 223
Annadale, E., 188, 219
antenatal
   check-ups, 87; ward, 26, 27, 51, 114, 118, 125
Apurbabari village, 9, 12, 15-8, 20, 29, 31-3, 63-4, 74, 76, 78, 81-3, 89, 91, 95, 97-8, 100, 102-3, 105-6, 111, 116, 125, 131, 139, 145, 155, 158, 169, 172, 175-8, 203-4
ayahs, 21, 23, 26, 28, 52, 90, 111, 114, 119, 127, 132-3, 138, 140, 153-5, 168; special, 10, 26, 52, 54, 108, 114, 119, 127-8, 153-5, 157, 209; silent sufferings of, 209
ayurvedic practices, 179
azan, 41
Aziz, K.M.A., 16, 228

Balachandran, I., 224
Bangladesh Bureau of Statistics (BBS), 5-6, 18, 23, 28, 193-4, 220
Bangladesh is a modern State, 199
Bangladesh Rural Advancement Committee (BRAC), 9, 19-20, 29, 131, 219, 221, 224; primary school, 19
Bangladeshi Government's policy to provide free health care, 192
baobatash, 78-80
Barfield, T., 178, 220
baribandh (closing house), 103-4
Barkat, A., 220
Barker, K.K., 184, 220
batash (evil wind), 42, 64
bazaar, 17
Becker, A., 220
Begum, S.F, 4, 226
Begum, T., 88, 226
Belle, A., 173, 175, 220
Bengali hospitality, 35
Bengali Muslim Society, 16
Bhatia, S , 220
Biesele, M., 108-9, 220
biomedical professionals, 121, 145, 162, 166, 171, 182-9, 197, 205-7, 212-3; communication of, 123; sensitising, 214
birth
   canal, 32, 40, 70, 84, 91-2, 98, 102, 116, 131, 144, 158, 174-5, 206; celebrating, 73; cleansing birth substances, 154; demedicalising, 213-4; events, 7, 9-10, 12, 29, 31, 33-4, 46, 63-6, 68, 70-1, 74, 85-7, 93, 95, 97-9, 117, 162, 164-6, 168-70, 172-3, 175,

184, 200, 204; hospital, 9, 10, 32, 46, 86-7, 105, 111, 117, 122, 131, 145, 157-9, 166-8, 171-3, 184-5, 187, 204, 213; impurity of, 51; meaning, 200; physiology of, 1; practices, 1-2, 4, 6-9, 11-2, 15, 31, 58-9, 63, 107, 109, 111, 122, 145, 157-8, 161, 173-6, 179-80, 186, 198, 200, 203-9, 211-2, 214, 216-7, 220-1; recognising women's active roles in, 203; skills of birth attendants, 9; trauma, 92

birthing
care, 1, 2, 7-8, 10, 32, 106, 169, 200, 203, 205, 216-7, 219; first birthing experience, 3; indigenous, 1, 5-7, 11, 31-2, 58, 89, 101, 173, 175, 201, 204, 209, 212; place, 38, 85, 94; posture, 70, 94; sharing their birthing experience, 37; stories, 11; woman's mother, 122

Biswas, S., 30, 109, 220
Blanchet, T., 1, 6-7, 16, 63, 108-9, 172, 174, 177, 221
Bloor, M., 186, 221
bodily mechanism, 65, 68-70, 87, 122, 167, 204
Bordo, S., 170, 221
Bose, M.L., 220
breast milk, 43
British period, 16
Broom, D.H., 168, 221
Browner, C., 221
Buddhism, 16, 17
buying medicine, 99, 132-3

caesarean, 4, 6, 27-8, 52, 54, 59, 126, 138-9, 142-3, 145, 148, 152, 160, 186, 193-5, 208-9, 213
Campbell, O.M.R., 4, 7, 227
Caplan, J., 225, 233
Carr, C.T, 171, 222
Carver, R., 198, 230
cervical injuries, 92
Chakravarty, J., 6, 220
Chatterjee, P., 169-70, 177, 195, 199, 201, 221
Chawla, J., 4, 86, 172, 178-9, 221
check-up room, 51, 53, 118

child mortality, 5
childbirth
complexities of, 161, 203; diversity of, 12; experiences, 4, 12, 122, 124, 162, 195, 200; situating, 203; writings, 3
Chin, V.V.P., 175, 232
chochi
afraid of, 76, touch of, 76
chodighar, 35
choditula ceremony, 51, 73, 102
Choudhury, B.R., 224
Chowdhury, A.M.R, 7, 109, 193, 221
Chowdhury, A.S., 7, 109, 193, 221
Chowdhury, M., 6, 108, 174, 224
Chowdhury, Z., 193-4, 221
chula, 18, 30, 34, 37, 41-3, 45, 70, 76-7
Clifford, J., 232
clinical assistant, 2, 3, 25, 28, 52, 141-4, 148
coconut oil, 48, 127
community health workers, 9, 12, 20, 66, 73, 87, 89, 155-6, 158
complicated cases, 98, 172
concealing of information, 126
Connor, L.H., 230
cord-cutting, 48, 93
corrupt practices, 159, 193-4, 201, 205, 207, 215
corruption, 193-4, 215, 227
Cosminsky, S., 109, 172-3, 175, 221
cosmopolitan
birthing system, 4; obstetric care, 5, 7-8, 31, 64, 97, 111, 113, 145, 161, 183, 191, 199-201, 204; obstetric service, 45; obstetrics, 1, 3-5, 11-2, 31, 112, 141, 157, 171-3, 176, 180, 183, 186, 196, 201, 203-5, 207-8, 216-7, 220
Cosslett, T., 166, 221
Costello, A., 138, 193, 229
Coulson, J., 171, 222
courage, 3, 37, 83, 87, 91, 96
Cousins, M., 185, 222
Coyaji, K.J., 183, 224
Cranny-Francis, A., 222

INDEX

Cross, A., 5, 220, 221, 222, 226-8, 231, 228
Cunnigham-Burley, S., 221, 230

dainis, 9, 11-12, 34, 39, 63-5, 68, 75, 86-97, 105, 157, 162, 164, 167-8, 172-81, 196, 200, 205-6, 210-1; skills of, 68, 87, 89, 96, 206, 208
dalals, 119-20
Das, V., 172, 222
Dasgupta, B., 30, 109, 220
Davis-Floyd, R.E., 111, 222
degovernmentalise the State, 215
Denzin, N.K., 8, 10, 220, 222, 224-5
Department of Public Health Engineering (DPHE), 23
Descartes, René, 166
Dilation and Curettage, 134
Directorate of Health, 25
discharge certificate, 57-8, 140-1, 143, 146
District Hospital (DH), 5, 7, 24, 118
doctors, 2-3, 10, 21-3, 25-8, 30, 46, 52, 54-5, 57-9, 106, 108, 111-3, 115-7, 119, 121-8, 131-7, 139-55, 157-60, 166, 171, 174-7, 179-83, 185, 187-94, 196, 200, 204-8, 213-4, 230; attitudes to patients, 187, 189; behaviour of, 131; enculturation of, 205; inappropriate behaviour of, 129; intern, 2, 3, 25-6, 28, 124, 132, 134-5, 140-4, 146-8, 152-4, 158, 191; intern doctor stole medicine, 130; male, 48, 51, 54, 116-7, 127-8, 144-5, 188, 213; mistakes of, 135; rivalry among, 149; skills of, 141
Doyal, L., 7, 168, 190, 193, 196-9, 210, 222
Drexler, B., 175, 232
Dreyfus, H., 223
drug stores, 22, 27
Dunn, F.L., 59-60, 222
Dutt, D., 194, 222

Eagle, D., 171, 222
Eaoton, R.M., 222
eclampsia
 antepartum, 45; room, 26, 113-4, 143, 159

education, 5, 16, 19, 29, 120, 132, 160, 189, 196, 199, 214, 216
Ehrenreich, B., 181, 190, 196, 222
Elahi, M.E., 174, 202, 219
emotional support, 68, 84, 86, 94, 107, 109, 154, 166-8, 205, 213
English, D., 30, 60, 123, 181, 190, 196, 220, 222
environment of distrust, 135
Essential Obstetric Care (EsOC), 4, 6, 20, 215-6
ethnographic data, 2
evil
 spirits, 6, 42, 64, 76, 79, 81, 103, 108, 208; wind, 64, 79, 101-3
examination table, 51-2
Expanded Program on Immunisation (EPI), 21

Faisal, A. J., 220
fakir (spiritual healer), 96, 101-2, 104
family planning, 6, 21, 30, 155, 181
Family Welfare Assistants (FWAs), 21, 155
Faruque, A.S.G., 6, 220
Favre-Saada, J., 179, 222
fear
 of death, 38, 82-3, 109; of getting polluted, 41
feminists, 2, 11
fertility behaviour, 170
field paraprofessional, 9, 12, 20, 87-8, 155-6
fieldwork, 9-11, 15, 17-8, 20-1, 23, 25, 33, 45-6, 51, 63, 72, 74, 76, 98, 111-2, 117, 119, 152, 193, 203
Fisher, S., 187, 189, 223
foetus pressing, 70
food taboos, 34, 81, 208
Foster, G.M., 163, 188, 223
Foucauldian perspectives, 170-1, 197
Foucault, M., 1, 11, 163, 169, 171, 182, 184-7, 191, 196, 199, 221-3, 231
Freidson, E., 188, 190, 223
Fromm, E., 169, 223

Gaines, A.D., 188, 224
Ganatra, B.R., 183, 223

Ganges River, 16
Gardner, K., 108, 224
Gaskin, I.M., 166, 224
Gay, J., 227
Gazi, R., 6-8, 108, 174, 224
gender relations, 7
Good, B.J., 13, 171, 224
Goodburn, E.A., 6, 108, 174, 224
Gordon, C., 223
gorvochul (baby's hair at birth), 76
Graham, H., 167, 224
Graham, W., 174, 224
Greenhalgh, S., 161
Guba, E.G., 8, 224
Gupta, A., 109, 224
Gupta, B., 179, 224

Hahn, R.A., 188, 224
Handwerker, W.P., 229, 231
Haque, Y.A., 99, 225
Harlow, S.D., 4, 7, 227
Hatcher, J., 230
healers, 12, 19-20, 40, 63, 96, 101, 108, 202, 221-2, 227, 230-2
Health and Population Sector Programme (HPSP), 6, 21, 228
health
  care, 2, 5, 7, 11, 16, 20, 59-60, 165, 182-3, 186, 192, 195-8, 204, 209-11, 214, 216-7, 220-1, 226, 229-31, 233; facilities, 5-6, 15, 20, 29, 118, 183, 197, 229; maternal, 1, 4-6, 8, 15, 112, 156, 195, 198-9, 209-11, 215-7, 219, 229, 231; planners, 2; practitioners, 20, 96, 101, 105-8, 191, 202
Hedrick-Wong, Y, 226
Helali, J., 220
Hindu Zamindars, 16
Hinduism, 15, 16, 17
Holden, P., 231
homeopathic medicine, 100, 105
homeopathy, 20, 96, 106
hospital, 3, 7-10, 12-3, 15, 20-8, 30-2, 37, 45-48, 50-53, 55-6, 58-60, 64, 66, 68, 71, 75, 86, 87, 93, 96-7, 104-5, 108, 111-23, 125-55, 157-9, 162-4, 166-9, 171-3, 175-7, 180, 181-94, 198, 201-2, 204-7, 209, 211-5, 217, 226; causes of hospital deaths, 209; *dalal*, 51, 119; drugstore, 134, 135-6; environment, 114, 116, 130, 182, 191, 198, 205, 207, 213-4; expenditures, 115, 134, 145, 154, 215; experiences while attending, 115; journey from home to, 117; management of, 25; obstetric care, 12, 45-6, 66, 68, 97, 116, 126, 130, 144, 181, 191, 198, 212, 217; obstetric practices in Bangladeshi, 175; procedures, 146, 154; re-organisation of hospital services, 212; smell of, 121-2; starting for, 115; teaching, 2, 24, 111; thana, 118; treatment, 59, 117, 134, 139, 158, 205, 211
Hossain, M., 5, 225
Hossain, N., 226
Hudson-Rodd, N., 189, 209, 225
Hunt, L., 168, 225
Hussain, A., 185, 222
Hutchison, L., 222
hydor (evil spirit), 42

iatrogenesis, 186, 188
Illich, I., 188, 196, 197, 225, 233
indigenous
  childbirth, 3-6, 63, 99; knowledge, 4, 7, 11, 58, 66, 69, 86, 145, 162, 172-3, 178-81, 200, 204-6, 208-9, 210-11, 216, 217; practices, 5, 63, 179, 181, 206
Irigaray, L., 168, 225
Islam, A., 1, 230
Islam, Ashrafi, 16
Islam, S., 5, 228

Jahan, F.A., 5, 226
Jahan, K., 6, 225
Jansick, V.J., 225
Jeffery, P.M., 170, 172, 177, 180-1, 193-4, 225
Jeffery, R., 170, 172, 177, 180-1, 193-4, 225
Jirojwong, S., 162, 225
job accountability, 215
Johnson, A.C., 190-1, 231

INDEX

Johnson, J.M., 8, 220
Johnson, T.M., 128
Johnstone, M.J., 190, 225
Jones, S., 225
Jordan, B., 1, 3-4, 8, 99, 109-11, 161, 163-4, 167-8, 172-3, 175-6, 180, 184-7, 211, 225-6
Juncker, T., 7-8, 226

kabiraj (herbalist), 96, 101-3
kajol, 43
Kakar, D.N., 176-7, 179, 226
Kanam, S.T., 4, 7, 197, 226
Karim, F., 224
Kaufert, P.A., 1, 4, 86, 184, 226, 229
Kay, M.A., 1, 109, 161, 172-3, 226
Keller, E.F., 228
Khan, A.K.Z., 174, 202, 219
Khan, A.R., 4, 219, 226
Khan, M.H., 7-8, 226
Khan, M.S.H., 4, 7, 145, 197, 226
Khanna, R., 224
Khanum, P.A., 1, 7, 8, 226, 230
Khuse, H., 188, 190, 226
Killingsworth, J.R, 193, 226, 231
Kitzinger, S., 1, 4, 109, 161-2, 168, 172-6, 184, 226-7
Kleinman, A., 8, 163-4, 222, 227
kneel down, 71
knowledge
    authoritative, 159, 167-8, 184-6, 197, 200-1, 204-5, 213, 220-2, 226-7, 231-223; cultural, 6, 16, 78, 84-5, 108; depending on *dainis*, 87; embodied, 3, 69, 124, 162, 165, 169, 184, 200, 205-6, 210, 213; experiential, 69, 86-8, 122, 181, 185; rationalist, 188, 191; sharing, 168
Koblinsky, M.A., 4, 7, 227
Kohli, S., 193, 222, 227
Konner, M., 188, 227
Kothari, M.L., 188, 191, 194-5, 227

laboratory tests, 24, 29, 118
labour
    bed, 27; pain, 2, 33-5, 37-9, 46, 52, 65, 69-70, 75, 82, 90, 94, 101-2, 116, 120, 122, 124, 157, 169; room, 10, 22, 26-7, 46-8, 54, 113-4, 118, 121-2, 124, 126-30, 142-4, 148-50, 153-5, 168, 213; table, 23, 47, 121, 124, 126-8, 130, 158, 213
Laderman, C., 172, 176, 227
Lawrence, J.V., 182, 227
Lazaraus, E., 187, 227
Leppard, M., 1, 7, 193, 227
Leslie, C., 59, 60, 222, 224, 227
library facilities, 26
life-threatening situations, 96
Lincoln, Y.S., 8, 220, 222, 224-5, 229
Lindenbaum, S., 179, 225-6, 227
literacy rate, 5, 19
local health practitioners, 20, 101, 105-8
Lock, M., 166, 222, 225-6, 228
Lyon, A., 170, 172, 177, 180-1, 193-4, 225

MacCormack, C.P., 1, 109, 161, 172, 221, 226, 228
Macintosh, J., 186, 221
Mahbub, A., 193, 221
Mahmud, S.N., 5, 109, 219
Maine, D., 183, 231
male attendants, 128, 131-3
malnourishment, 5, 12, 139, 166
Maloney, C., 16, 228
Manderson, L., 225
Mannan, I., 174, 202, 219
Marcus, G.E., 232
Margarita, A., 226-7, 231
Marshall, T., 174, 224
Martin, E., 4, 111, 161, 171, 184, 186, 188, 228-9
massaging limbs, 84
massaging oil, 71, 91, 173
Maternal and Child Welfare Centres (MCWCs), 5-6
maternal
    morbidity, 4, 208, 224; mortality, 4-5, 28, 183, 197-01, 224, 229, 231-3
maternity wards, 2
McClain, C.S., 231
McHugh, S. 227

Mckeganey, N.P., 221, 230
McKeown, T., 228, 199
Medical College Hospital (MCH), 2, 5-6, 9, 12, 15, 20, 22, 24-5, 28-9, 31, 45, 51, 53, 58-9, 111-3, 117-8, 126-7, 133-4, 137-9, 141, 145-6, 152-3, 157, 194, 203-4, 213
medical bureaucracies, 209
medicine list, 47, 52, 134-5, 143, 146, 151
Mehta, L.A., 188, 191, 194-5, 227
membrane ruptured, 92
menstruation, 33, 69
mental strength, 35, 65-6, 68, 83-4, 102, 165, 204
methodology, 11, 219
midwifery, 165-7, 178, 196, 214, 220
Miers, M., 230
Miller, P., 223
Ministry of Finance, 5, 198-9, 228
Ministry of Health and Family Welfare (MOHFW), 1, 4-7, 13, 21, 180, 196, 228
Mishler, E.G., 187, 228
Mitra, S.N., 5, 228
moner shahosh (mental strength), 35, 64-6, 68, 70, 83-4, 107, 122, 165, 204
Mostafa, G., 225
Mughal regime, 16
murubbis (elders), 81

Nahar, S., 4, 7, 138, 145, 193, 197, 226, 229
Nandy, A., 169, 170, 184, 227-8
Nasrin, T., 4, 7, 145, 197, 226
National Health Service (NHS), 193
National Institute for Population Research and Training (NIPORT), 3-4, 7, 228-9
nausea, 69
Navarro, V., 196, 198-9, 229
Newman, L.A., 175, 232
Nissim, R., 224
Non-Governmental Organisations (NGOs), 1, 5, 198, 211-2, 215-6; paraprofessionals, 6; run health program, 66; services, 19

normal vaginal delivery, 139
nurse/(s), 10, 21-3, 25-7, 46-8, 50-1, 54, 57-9, 90, 108, 111, 114-6, 119, 122-7, 129-33, 135-40, 143, 145-6, 148-55, 157-9, 166, 171, 174-7, 185, 187-91, 193-4, 196, 200, 204-8, 213-5, 222, 225; attitudes of, 151; attitudes to patients, 150, 187; In-charge, 115, 134, 143-4, 150-52; seniority of, 152; staff, 25, 150; student, 25, 28, 149, 150, 152, 153, 191
Nursing Institution, 25, 152
Nursing Superintendent, 25
Nursing Supervisor, 150

Oakley, A., 4, 8, 111, 162-3, 167, 171, 183-4, 186-8, 197, 224, 229
observational experiences, 12, 29, 58, 63, 107, 206
obstetric care, 2, 5, 7-8, 11, 15, 20, 24, 31, 64, 97, 111-13, 134, 145, 149, 155, 157, 161-2, 164-5, 181, 183, 186, 191, 194, 197, 199-01, 204, 207, 212-3, 216, 220, 224-26, 229-30, 232
obstetrical practices, 4
occupational pattern, 18, 29
ojha (snakebite healer), 96
Olsen, V., 10, 229
operating theatre, 26-8, 54, 114, 118, 134, 142-3, 149-50
Ottawa Charter, 210, 212, 215

panipora, 102-3
Patel, T., 229
Paul, B.K., 182, 224, 229
personal care, 83, 152
Peters, C.J., 175, 232
pharmaceutical representatives, 135, 158
Phillips, D.R., 182-3, 193, 198, 229
physical
    energy, 68, 105-6, 159; supports, 84, 94, 175; vigour, 65-6, 83
pirs, 16
placenta was usually buried, 95
policy-makers, 2
pollution *(napak)*, 44, 102; birth, 3, 6, 76, 177-8, 231; ritual, 76, 177; stink of, 177

Porter, M., 187, 189, 229
Porter, S., 190, 230
postnatal wards, 26, 113-4, 126
pregnancy
 kol-bekol (problems in pregnancy), 37, 64, 68; first, 34; rate, 20; *silence during*, 204
Press, N., 221
Price, J., 221, 226
privacy
 is infringed, 176; lack of, 158; maintaining, 125
private practice, 119, 138, 142
psychological
 isolation, 121, 166; sufferings, 166, 194, 200
push down, 40, 48, 66, 90, 92, 121

Quaiyum, M. A., 1, 230
quilts, 39, 42-3, 82

Rabinow, P., 223
Rahman, A., 226
Rahman, A.P.M.S., 4, 7, 145, 197, 226
Rahman, M., 106
Rahman, M.H., 174, 202, 219
Ram, K., 4, 172, 179-81, 230
Rao, V.N., 183, 224
Rashid, S.F., 1, 6-8, 63, 159, 162, 172, 219
recite surahs from the *Koran*, 68
relationships between nurses and doctors, 152, 187
remaining silent, 120
research results, 205
Residential Medical Officer (RMO), 21, 23, 46, 48, 133
resuscitate the baby, 48, 54, 124
resuscitation, 50, 121
Reynolds, P.C., 163, 230
Rice, P.L., 225
Richman, J., 188-9, 230
rituals of cleansing, 45
Rose-Ackerman, S., 193, 230

Rothman, B.K., 1, 4, 161, 165-7, 171, 175, 184-5, 188, 230
Rozario, S., 1, 6, 16-7, 63, 108-10, 172, 174, 177, 221, 230, 232

Safe Motherhood Initiatives (SMIs), 6-8, 131, 180, 196, 207, 215-6
Saha, T, 5, 228
saline drip, 47, 54, 57
Samuel, G., 108, 221, 230, 232
Sanders, D., 198, 230
sanitation, 19
Sargent, C.F., 1, 4, 108-9, 172, 178, 184, 220-22, 226-8, 231-2
Sarker, P., 16, 228
Sawicki, J., 171, 231
Scheper-Hughes, N., 166, 228
Schulz, R., 190-91, 231
Sengupta, S., 30, 109, 220
Sesia, P.M.,163, 168, 231
Shaiken, H., 225, 233
shameless, 74
sharam, 39, 41, 60, 73-6, 83, 89, 98-9, 107, 117-8, 129, 169-70, 204-5, 208; issue of, 117; matter of, 39, 73, 76, 83, 98, 107, 117
Shasthya Kormi (SK), 155, 160
shaving hair, 60, 73
Shi, L., 199, 229
Shildrick, M., 221
shoriler shakti, 64-6, 68, 70, 84, 107, 122, 165, 204
Shostak, M., 108, 231
Shuttleworth, S., 228
sitting down posture, 71
Smith, D.E., 161, 231
Somjee, G., 177, 179-80, 231
squatting position, 71
sterilising instruments, 126
stomach cramps, 39
suffer silently, 170, 205
Sufi-oriented Islam, 16
Sundari, T.K., 183, 231
support of men, 99

tabiz (amulets), 96, 101-4
tending patients, 131, 154
Teresa, Mother, 146, 160
Tew, M., 4, 8, 195, 231
Thaddeus, S., 183, 231
Thana Family Planning Officer (TFPO), 21, 30
Thana Health Complex (THC), 6, 9, 12, 15, 20-24, 29-31, 39, 46-8, 51-2, 55, 58-9, 66, 73, 90, 97, 111, 115-7, 122-3, 127, 130, 133, 138-9, 144, 152, 156-7, 192, 203, 212; annual budget for, 24; upgrading of, 213
Thomas, S., 226, 231
Timyan, J., 227
Traditional Birth Attendants (TBAs), 5-7, 9, 20, 88, 112-3, 144, 180, 202, 219; training program, 88, 174, 180
traditional midwifery, 196
transparency of decisions, 215
Trevanthan, W. R., 175, 232
Turner, B.S., 181-2, 190, 193, 232
Tyler, S.A., 232

UNICEF, 6-7, 180, 225, 232-3
Union Health and Family Welfare Centre (UHFWC), 5-6, 20
Unnithan-Kumar, M., 172, 232

Vallis, T.M., 227
van Alten, D., 212, 232
van Mannen, J., 8, 232
Verhasselt, Y., 193, 230
Vincent, P., 224
violence
  fiscal, 162, 191; causes fiscal, 209
Vivoni-Farge, E., 182, 232

Vlassoff, C., 230
vomiting, 41, 69, 93, 109

Wagner, M., 112, 159, 162-3, 175, 196, 214, 232
Walker, R., 225
Weedon, C., 163-4, 170, 232
Whitford, M., 225
Whittaker, A., 186, 233
Wilkinson, G., 230
Wilsford, D., 193, 233
woman
  are silent, 169; blessing birthing, 91; deprived of the social facilities, 199; doctor harassed, 140; empowering, 11, 210; felt degraded and intimidated, 129; in Africa, 3; interests of, 11; labouring, 2; poor, 1-2, 5, 8, 11, 31-2, 46, 61, 101, 158, 172, 181-3, 185, 187-8, 191-2, 194-5, 200-01, 203-7, 212, 216-7; pregnant women's husbands, 105; pregnant, 2, 4, 20, 30, 69, 82, 87-8, 101, 105, 118, 155-6, 158, 225, 229; rural women in Bangladesh, 12, 161-2; rural, 1, 3, 6-7, 12, 31, 55, 60, 64-5, 73-4, 78, 83-4, 91, 101-2, 105, 107-8, 111, 114, 117-8, 122-6, 129-31, 145, 156, 158-9, 161-4, 166-73, 179-82, 184-8, 191, 194-5, 197, 199, 200, 206, 208, 210-11, 213-4, 216, 219; rural women's versions, 186; silent, 158
World Bank Reports, 5, 7-8
World Health Organisation (WHO), 174, 180, 196, 210, 212, 215-6, 233

York, G., 186, 233

Zola, I.K., 185, 194, 219, 222, 225-6, 230, 233